Fitness is Sexy

A Different Approach

By: Sandra Hampton

9781635010466

PUBLISHERS NOTES

Disclaimer – Speedy Publishing LLC

This publication is intended to provide helpful and informative material. It is not intended to diagnose, treat, cure, or prevent any health problem or condition, nor is intended to replace the advice of a physician. No action should be taken solely on the contents of this book. Always consult your physician or qualified health-care professional on any matters regarding your health and before adopting any suggestions in this book or drawing inferences from it.

The author and publisher specifically disclaim all responsibility for any liability, loss or risk, personal or otherwise, which is incurred as a consequence, directly or indirectly, from the use or application of any contents of this book.

Any and all product names referenced within this book are the trademarks of their respective owners. None of these owners have sponsored, authorized, endorsed, or approved this book.

Always read all information provided by the manufacturers' product labels before using their products. The author and publisher are not responsible for claims made by manufacturers.

This book was originally printed before 2014. This is an adapted reprint by Speedy Publishing LLC with newly updated content designed to help readers with much more accurate and timely information and data.

Speedy Publishing LLC

40 E Main Street, Newark, Delaware, 19711

Contact Us: 1-888-248-4521

Website: http://www.speedypublishing.co

REPRINTED Paperback Edition: ISBN: 9781635010466

Manufactured in the United States of America

DEDICATION

I dedicate this book to my family and to everyone who desires to live a healthy lifestyle.

TABLE OF CONTENTS

Chapter 1- First Things First

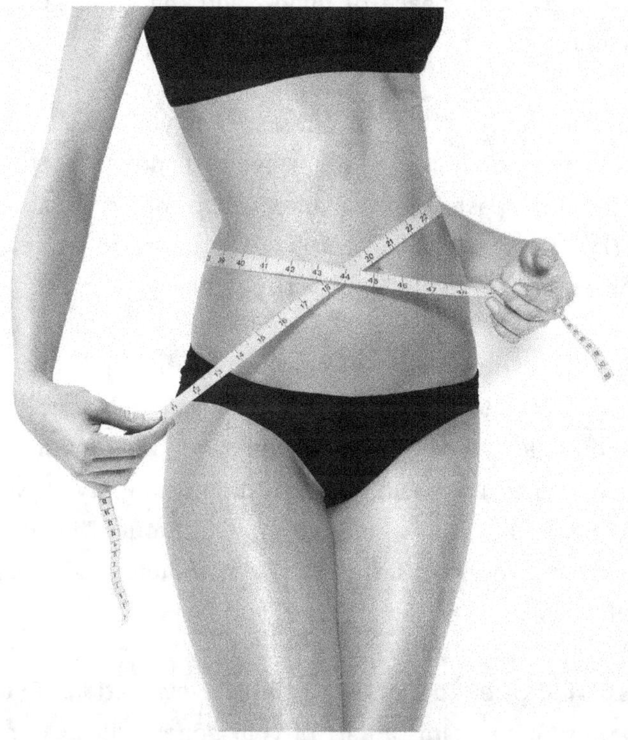

There is one common mistake which many people make when they decide to improve their bodies. This mistake is to not begin with adequate preparation. The first, and most essential, step in preparing to embark on a home workout program is to have a complete health clearance from your physician.

The most important reason for this is you may have a medical problem which you do not know exists. There are many health conditions which can worsen from strenuous exercise; there are some which can even be fatal. While you want to work toward that perfect body, you surely do not want to take unnecessary chances with your health or your life.

An evaluation from your physician will allow you to see if you have any extraordinary risk factors. This kind of check-up, which will take very little time or cost, is well worth the benefits. A clean bill of health will give you peace of mind-- and the go-ahead for your home work out.

The second reason is to find out whether you have any special limitations. For example, you may have had sprains or other types of injuries in the past. These can affect choosing the home workout that is right for you. Your doctor may advise you to modify certain kinds of exercise, or to avoid them altogether.

Visiting your physician before you begin a home workout regimen is necessary. If you have any health or medical problems, they need to be addressed before you start a home workout. Anything from a prior injury to an unknown heart condition can prevent you from getting the results you want from your workout. They can cause setbacks, and even disaster. A few minutes of your time beforehand can prevent all of this.

The best kind of evaluation is a complete evaluation. If you have not made routine exams a part of your general lifestyle, now is a good time to start. When you are serious about beginning a home workout regimen, you probably already know that it will affect your body. Whether you have exercised before or not, making a home work out a part of your everyday life will place stress and strain on your body.

It will affect your muscles, your joints, your blood pressure, and every other part of your system. Your body will be working much harder than it ever did before, to move in the direction of your goals. This is why you need to know in advance that your body is ready for the task. It will help your workouts to proceed more smoothly, and without any unnecessary risks to your health.

A home workout is an exciting adventure. However, in addition to the effects it will have on your body, it will also affect your mind. From the increased blood flow which occurs during workouts, to the change in your blood-sugar levels, the physical benefits of exercise can affect your mood, spirits, and disposition. In order to ensure that these changes are positive and you gain as much from them as possible, you need to be prepared by knowing that you are healthy.

Many people have sustained permanent injuries, and worse, solely due to not being aware of medical problems or limiting conditions prior to starting a regimen of strenuous exercise. Others have become overwhelmed and discouraged, leading them to quit before seeing any positive results. Still others have given up, because they simply did not know what to expect from their new venture. In most cases, all of these repercussions can be avoided.

You want your new home workout routine to produce great results. You want the perfect body that you may have been dreaming of for many years. You want it all to come in the healthiest, safest, and most enjoyable manner, without any unnecessary risks or setbacks. Getting a complete evaluation from your doctor before you choose any exercise or purchase any equipment is the best way to make your home workout routine a positive experience.

When you know that you are healthy, and without any risk factors, you will have a double benefit. First, you can take on the workout routines of your choice without undue risk to your health; and second, you will have the peace of mind from knowing that your new venture is safe for you.

In the interest of your health and safety, make an appointment to see your doctor before you begin your new home workout. Not only is this the most sensible step, it will do wonders for your self-confidence. When you know that you are physically prepared for the home workout routines which you are about to begin, you can look forward to one of the best and most exciting experiences of your life.

Making a Plan

The second mistake many people make when starting a home workout is to not make a plan in advance. They buy expensive equipment which they really do not need, or believe that they must do certain kinds of exercises which they truly dislike. While many make this mistake because they believe that whatever is currently popular is the method they must try, others do not realize that a home workout is meant to be fun! You can avoid both of these mistakes by making a workout plan that is right for you.

The first point to consider is what you, yourself, enjoy. If you do not choose routines which you enjoy doing, you might dislike it so much that you quit. You may force yourself to continue doing them, while hating every minute of it. Instead, by focusing on the types of routines which interest you the most, you will be well-motivated each time you do your routines, enjoy them much more, and move closer and closer to your goals.

The second point to think about is your own particular needs. While this will be discussed further in later chapters, it is something which you should consider. Is your main priority to develop "six-pack" abs, to change a flabby body into lean muscle, or to gain overall strength? When you address your goals, it will be easier to choose the workout which focuses on these goals.

The third point is expense. While you may be thinking of a home work out as a less-costly alternative to joining a gym or hiring a personal trainer, if you are tempted to buy all of the latest home exercise equipment you may be dismayed to find that these costs are even higher. When you decide on the equipment that is necessary for your home work out, you can keep the expense at a minimum. You may even decide that you do not need to purchase any equipment at all.

There is another, equally-important reason for making a plan before you begin. Making a plan also gives you control of your home work out experience. If you think about it, this is true about anything worthwhile in life. If you begin something without first putting some careful thought into planning, you can end up with an entire course of action that is not suitable for you. You may feel overwhelmed, exhausted, discouraged, and confused. You might not even be sure if you are making any real progress.

Making a plan will eliminate all of these worries and give you the home workout routine that you will love to do on a regular basis. You will be more satisfied with the results, and happier with yourself.

How do you go about making a home workout plan? You can begin by setting goals which include reasonable expectations. If you want that perfect body, you can have it-- but you cannot have it overnight! You also cannot have it without work! When you set your goals, and include reasonable expectations about how much work you will need to do and how long it should take for you to see results, this is the foundation of a good plan.

A good plan also includes some leeway for error. For example, you may choose a specific exercise, but soon discover that it is not right for you. Even if you give it your best effort, you may find that it causes too much pain or discomfort, or places too much emphasis on a certain part of the body. When you are making your home work out plan, allowing room for error can eliminate frustration. You will not have an unnecessary sense of failure if this is included in your plan.

A good plan must be reasonable about the amount of time you can devote to your home workouts. As no one these days has unlimited time, it is important to not commit yourself to working out for many hours each day when you cannot fit such a regimen into your daily schedule. Not only would it make your workouts a burden, it would interfere with the rest of your day's priorities. You would end up too tired to do your job, or to enjoy quality time with your family.

However, you also cannot afford to make your home workouts the lowest subject on your priority list. Logically, if you do a workout only when you feel like it, or only when it is convenient, you will not obtain the results you want. Your plan should reflect the amount of time you can put into your workouts on a regular basis, and make a point of adhering to it. No matter how busy your life may be, you can make an appropriate amount of time for your workouts.

One way to do this is to assess your everyday schedule, and decide on the best time for your workouts. Whether this means getting up a little earlier so that you can work out before you go to school or to your job, or using half of your lunch hour to work out, it should be easy to fit your workouts into your schedule without disrupting your everyday life.

Making an advance plan will keep the chaos, confusion, and frustration out of your home workouts. You will know what you need to do, and when you need to do it. You will have a general idea of what kind of results you can expect to see, and how long it will take before they occur. When you add all of these factors together, your home work out will be something for you to look forward to, each and every time!

Exercises

If you want that perfect body you have always dreamed of, you will need to exercise! The good news is that exercising does not have to mean boring routines which can soon become tiresome. There are three categories of exercises which will help you to gain that perfect body. When you have some information about each type, you can choose from amongst them to custom-design a home work out to meet your needs and personal preferences.

One form of exercise is known as pilates. While pilates have become increasingly popular during the last few years, it is not a modern concept at all. The basic principles of pilates go back as far as World War One, when they were developed in Germany by Joseph Pilate.

These exercise routines are great for the overall body, while placing much emphasis on the areas which most people find to be trouble-spots. Whether you are hoping to lose unwanted fat, or develop as much healthy muscle as possible, pilates are an excellent choice for your home workout routine. Your abs, hips, buttocks, and thighs will all benefit from pilates. Your muscles will become stronger, more flexible, and healthier.

There are many different exercise routines in the pilates category. Some of the most popular are "the Hundred" and "the Roll-Up," which will do wonders for your abdominal muscles; and "the Single-Leg Stretch" and "the Double-Leg Stretch," which will tone your buttocks and hips as well as your abdominal region. Many of the pilates exercises do not require any kind of exercise equipment other than a basic mat.

Aerobics is another popular form of exercise. While aerobics routines will assist in toning your muscles, there is a more important reason for including aerobics in your home work out. Aerobics will benefit your entire cardiovascular system. When you are thinking about that perfect body, health is as important as appearance. Adding aerobics exercise to your workout routine will strengthen your heart and your lungs. It will promote better health, as well as making your workout a truly exhilarating experience.

Calisthenics may already be familiar to you. You may remember some calisthenics exercises from your school days. However, you may not have known how beneficial they can be in helping you to create the body of your dreams. Whether or not you enjoyed calisthenics as a youngster, they will go a long way in sculpting that perfect body.

There are many different calisthenics exercises from which to choose, so you can easily incorporate some of your favorites into your home work out. Some of the most common calisthenics exercises are jumping jacks, abdominal crunches, push-ups, sit-ups, and squats. They will get your blood pumping, and tone and firm your body. It will be fun to see how exercises you learned as a child can be so useful in helping you to create the perfect body you want today.

When you have custom-designed the exercise routines you wish to include in your home work out, you are partway to developing the workout which you will do each session. However, there are a couple of other points to consider before your workout regimen is complete. These extra points will make your workouts less stressful on your body.

First, regardless of the types of exercises you have chosen, you must begin each session with a warm-up. A brief period of basic stretching and bending will give your body the preparation it needs to be ready for a workout. This little preliminary can make quite a difference. When your body is readied beforehand, the exercising will flow more naturally and smoothly.

Second, a cooling-down period should be at the end of every home workout. The same kinds of stretching and bending motions that you used to warm up will help your body to conclude the workout. It will prepare your body for rest.

It is not difficult to choose the forms of exercise that are best for you. You can start by thinking about the types of exercise you like the most, and confirm to them your specific needs. You can tone the areas which are most in need of attention, or aim for an overall workout which will benefit your entire body.

It is important to choose exercises which you will not tire of, so that you will be motivated to do your workout on a regular basis. If you keep your expectations reasonable, and demonstrate self-discipline, you will be pleased with the results. You can begin to see your body's shape and strength improve within a relatively short period of time. The perfect body you have always wanted can be yours-- and it all starts with custom-designing your own exercise routine.

Chapter 2- Getting Fit Weight Lifting

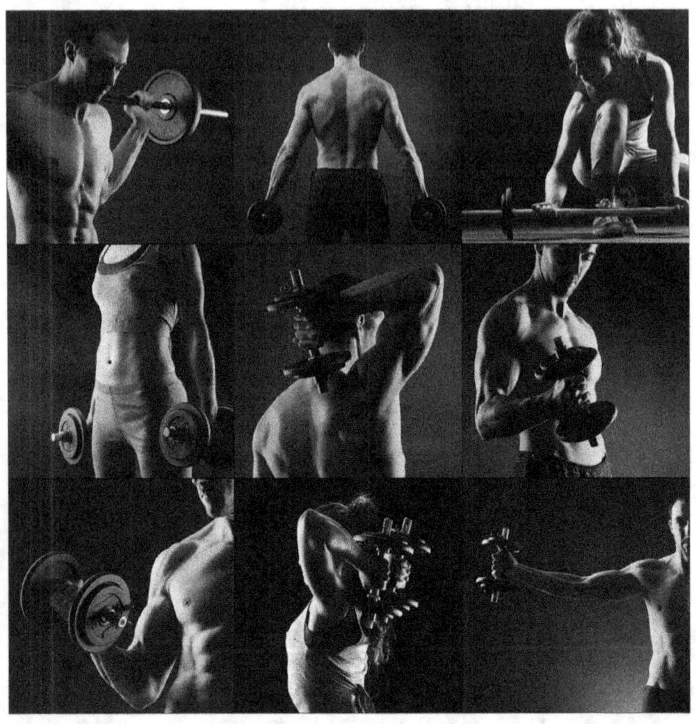

When you think of gaining that perfect body, thoughts of weights may come to mind. Whether this is positive or negative depends on your opinion. While planning a great home workout can include the use of weights, a workout can be done without them. In addition, there are a number of different kinds of weights, if you do decide to use them.

One form of weights is known as dumbbells. These are good to use when doing exercises while standing. While dumbbells can greatly tone the muscles in your arms, shoulders, and upper torso, they can also assist in toning your abdominal muscles.

Dumbbells can be found in a variety of different weights. When you are beginning your workouts, it is a good idea to start with lighter dumbbell, and increase the weight as your body becomes accustomed to the workouts.

A second form of weights is barbells. They are generally used while lying flat. While the power exercise known as bench-pressing is popular amongst professional body-builders and other athletes, you can easily make it a part of your own home workout routine. As bench-pressing places a considerable amount of strain on the body, especially the abdomen, it is essential to choose light weights when you are beginning your workout routines. Otherwise, this strain could cause permanent damage to your muscles. When you choose lighter weights, you can easily work up to heavier weights as your body becomes accustomed to this practice.

While dumbbells and barbells are available in various weights, there is an additional feature which can be useful to you. Dumbbells and barbells are both available in a solid, one-piece style, and in a style which allows you to take off and add on weights as your needs change. The latter can be the most beneficial to your workout routine, as you can continue to adjust the amount of weight you use to reflect the progress you make in your workouts.

You may also be wondering if you can get that perfect body without using any weights at all. The answer to this is yes, it is possible, but it is likely to take longer. The exercises you do with weights direct the focus to specific points in your body. The use of the weights helps these points to tone and strengthen quicker and easier. Power exercises done with weights will give you that perfect body faster, but this does not mean you cannot get the body you want without using them. If you are prepared to work harder and longer, you can reach your goal without using weights.

If you have decided that weights are a good addition to your home work out, there are some safety tips to make your workout better, more pleasurable, and without undue risk. Please do not simply order weights and begin using them without considering these tips first.

One tip is to be sure you choose the right weights. If you are not accustomed to using this kind of workout equipment, it cannot be stressed too strongly that you should select light weights. Whether you are considering barbells, dumbbells, or both, you do not want to put too much strain on your body and risk injury.

Another tip is to ensure your safety when you work out with weights. While this is true for exercising in general, maneuvering weights in a standing position means wearing appropriate workout gear. You should have sneakers or similar shoes with non-slip rubber soles. You should also avoid wearing clothes that are too loose or long sleeves.

It is also important to be sure that you are working out on a safe floor. Slipping or falling can be especially dangerous if you are working out with weights. You should avoid floors with rugs, carpeting, tile, and other potentially hazardous material or coverings. Whether you create your own home gym, or simply devote one particular part of your home to a workout space, you must keep your safety in mind when you work out with your weights.

Working out with weights can give you that perfect body! It will also invigorate your entire system. Your heart and lungs will greatly benefit when you make working out with weights a part of your home workout routine. If you keep all of these tips in mind, start slowly, and do not demand overnight results, you will be amazed at how quickly you do begin to see results.

Your body will not only feel stronger, it will actually be stronger. The new tone you will see in your muscles will be beyond compare. That perfect body you have always dreamed of will be more than just a dream-- it will start to take shape, and be in the best condition of your life.

What About Other Equipment?

One mistake many people make when preparing to do home workouts is to go overboard in purchasing exercise equipment. They end up wasting money on expensive equipment they do not really need, and cluttering their homes with products they will not use. When you are preparing to do home workouts, some tips will help you to decide what kinds of equipment are suitable for you.

One point to consider is the amount of space you have in the area where you plan to work out. A good rule of thumb is that you probably do not need more equipment than you can comfortably fit in that space. Even the smallest workout space can accommodate your exercise equipment if you do not purchase unnecessary products.

A second factor is cost. While you may be tempted to purchase all of the popular equipment you have seen advertised, the expense is rarely worth it. You do not have to equip your workout space to rival a gymnasium-- you can have that great body without it.

The third factor is your goal. As you probably already know what you hope to accomplish from your home workouts, selecting the right equipment will help you to reach your goal.

You should also consider your own preferences. If you are like most people, there are certain things which you like and certain things which you dislike. Even if you think specific types of exercise equipment are absolutely necessary, they will not get much use if you hate to use them. When you focus on your preferences, you will be more likely to get the exercise equipment that is best suited to you.

While taking these factors into consideration can assist you in choosing the right exercise equipment, there are a few types of equipment which are especially beneficial to the person who is beginning a new home workout regimen. With a little comparison-shopping, you can find them at a relatively low price to fit your budget. It is not necessary to buy name brands, or the most expensive model on the market. You can be price-conscious, while giving your new home work out the boost it needs to be successful and fun!

One piece of exercise equipment that is easy to use, enjoyable, and beneficial, is a stationary bike. A stationary bike can be the ideal way to warm up before your regular workout, or a nice change as a mini-workout in itself. A good stationary bike is adjustable, so that it will feel custom-fit for your personal comfort. It will provide all of the benefits of riding a bicycle-- right in your own home. It is a great way to exercise in general, as well as to focus on those troublesome spots. If you use a stationary bike on a regular basis, it will help to firm your hips, buttocks, and thighs. This is one type of exercise equipment that will make working out feel like play.

A treadmill will also provide special benefits. If you are new to working out, using a treadmill can help to increase your physical endurance. You will become able to breathe better, and gain better strength in your heart and lungs. As a perfect body has as much to do with increasing your health to its very best as it do with your appearance, a treadmill should be on your must-have list of home exercise equipment.

A rowing machine is another popular piece of exercise equipment. When your goal is that perfect body, you will be delighted with how quickly the regular use of a rowing machine begins to tone your abdominal muscles, your arms, and your shoulders. Not only will a rowing machine help to strengthen your upper body, it will increase your body's firmness. Your upper body will start to take on a better shape as your muscles become more well-defined.

If you have a large area of your home to devote to your workouts, and plenty of money to spare, you can choose a number of other types of exercise equipment for your workouts. However, you can have the best possible start to that perfect body without spending a lot of money or using a lot of space. When you begin your new home workouts with only these three pieces of exercise equipment, you may soon decide that you do not really need any others.

In addition, considering basic home exercise equipment as a worthwhile investment is a positive way to look at it. When you purchase these products, you are not only taking the first step toward creating the body of your dreams, you are also making strides toward a healthier body that can last for a lifetime. Even if you have only a small amount of money to put into your home workouts, these few pieces of exercise equipment will be well worth the investment. They will help you to reach your goal of a great-looking body, while increasing your overall health at the same time.

Do You Need More?

You may be well-motivated and looking forward to beginning your new home workout regimen. At the same time, you may be wondering if you could benefit from something more. You may be unsure of whether you are completely prepared to do it all on your own. If you think that you need a little extra help, it could very well put you on the right track.

One possibility is to enlist the aid of a personal trainer. It is not necessary to have a personal trainer at your side for the duration of your workouts-- some input when you are starting out can be very beneficial.

A personal trainer can help to customize your home workout regimen, if you are uncertain of what is right for you. He can also advise you of what to expect from your workouts. If you do not know how to deal with discomfort in your muscles, or how long you can reasonably expect to wait before you see results, a personal fitness trainer can answer all of your questions.

A second possibility is a short-term membership at a gym. Even if you plan to do your workouts in your own home, there is much to be gained from a few visits to a gym. You can see workout equipment in use, which can help you to decide which types of equipment you want for your home. You can interact with others who are working out, which will help you to see what you yourself need to do, and the results which you can expect. You can take this entire knowledge home with you, to put to use in your own workouts.

Another possible extra is for your home workouts to utilize the buddy system. While some people do very well at any venture on their own, others do much better if they are in the company of likeminded friends, or even family members. If you are in the latter category, encouraging others to join you in your home workouts can be useful to both you and the others in your life. Mutual support can be quite motivating. Even healthy, good-spirited competition can make your workouts more enjoyable and more oriented toward results.

The buddy system is not for everyone. There are many who do much better with working out alone. You probably already know which category describes you the best. Whichever one you choose, it should be the method that works for you.

An additional factor is your own level of motivation. There are many people who want great results, but are not sure that they have what it takes to get there. You may wonder if you will always have the time to devote to your workouts, or if you might become tired or discouraged and tempted to quit, or whether you may decide that it really is not worth the effort. If you want your home workout routine to be a success, and to give you that perfect body, it is a good idea to address these concerns in advance.

Everyone becomes discouraged at times, and no one is one-hundred-percent motivated each and every day. For your workouts to be a success, without the worry of quitting before you reach your goal, you should have a plan for how to deal with those less-than-ideal days before they occur.

As each person has his own method of getting things done, consider the method that works for you. How do you prime yourself to do something when you really do not feel like doing it? It could be a task at work, a household chore, or even something you usually like. No one is at his best every single day, but this does not mean you can afford to neglect whatever you must do. This includes your home work out routines.

When you know the method you use in your everyday life, you can apply the same methods to your workouts. Perhaps it involves getting yourself in a certain frame of mind. Perhaps you might give yourself a small treat, chat with a friend, or promise yourself a reward for a job well done. Whatever works for you, to help you to be motivated when you do not feel motivated at all, can be a wonderful aid to keeping you on track. If you have such a plan in advance, you will be less likely to skip your workouts, and more enthusiastic about doing them.

You may decide that you do not need any of these little "extras" at all. You may be the type of person who can commit a specific period of time into your daily schedule for workouts, and stick to it on a regular basis, without fail. If this sounds accurate, good for you! However, giving yourself the option for extra help when you need it is not a sign of weakness. It only means that you know yourself well enough to be aware that you may require a bit of extra help to be consistent with your home workouts. If it will help you to stay on the right track, incorporating some extra help into your basic workout plan is a positive step. It can keep you on the track toward success!

Chapter 3- Home Fitness Workout for Her

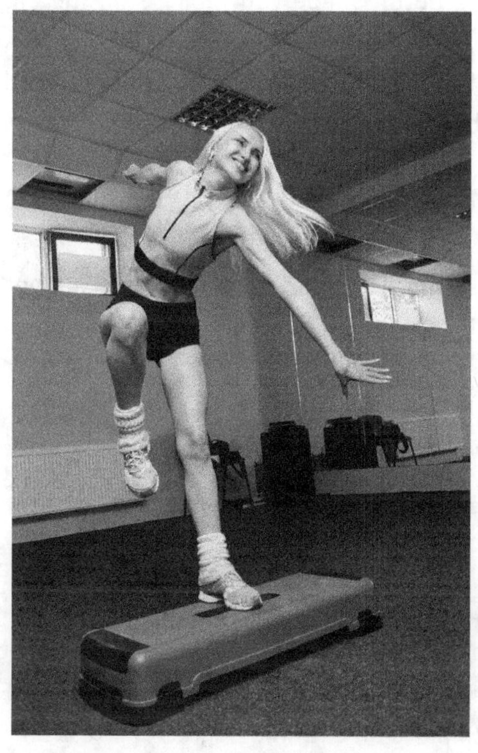

These days, home workouts are as popular amongst women as they are for men. Women have a natural desire to look and feel their best, too. This is evident by the large number of women who join gyms, purchase exercise equipment, and try various diets. While being more physically attractive and healthier are sensible goals for women, women who wish to begin home workouts do have special circumstances.

One topic is working out during pregnancy. You may have heard "old wives' tales" who claim that no exercise at all is safe when you are pregnant, and you may also heard that virtually nothing is off limits. If you are pregnant, or planning to become pregnant, you may be unsure of which point of view to believe.

Fitness is Sexy

With your doctor's approval, working out during pregnancy can be very beneficial. In fact, starting a home workout routine prior to becoming pregnant can prepare your body for this exciting adventure. The better shape your body is in, the easier and more comfortable your pregnancy and childbirth will be for you. It will also make returning to your pre-pregnant state easier and faster after your baby is born.

However, you should be sensible about your home workouts. Your goal is to get your body in its ideal condition, not to overtax your strength or put unreasonable demands on your body. The home workout routine you choose should reflect making your body stronger and more limber, and improving your muscle tone. It is unwise to go to extremes with working out while you are pregnant. If you really want to lift weights, it is best to wait until after your baby is born!

A second topic involves the female anatomy in general. Even when pregnancy is not an issue, you must still take this into consideration. Although it should be obvious, your body is made differently than that of your husband or brother. First, workout routines which place an extreme degree of stress on the abdominal and pelvic regions can indeed cause damage to the internal organs. This is something to keep in mind when you are choosing your home workout program.

In addition, the female muscles are not as prepared for strenuous routines as those of a man's. This does not mean that you cannot obtain the perfect body you want. It does mean taking on less, especially at the beginning, and proceeding slower. If working out is new to you, it is not a good idea to risk tearing muscles by attempting to do too much, too soon.

Whether your body is petite or full-figured, athletic or out of shape, you can have the perfect body of your dreams. In order to avoid the risk of unnecessary injuries, common sense is the key. After all, the purpose of working out is to get your body in its best possible shape, not to incur damage which can slow you down or even become permanent.

The woman who does not have pregnancy as a factor should assess her personal situation before planning a home workout routine. The current condition of your body, and how familiar it is with exercise in general, are two points to consider. If you are already athletic, and used to a moderate amount of exercise on a regular basis, you have more leeway than the woman who has never exercised and is quite out of shape.

Thinking about your goals is a positive way to begin. Do you want to increase your overall health, stamina, and be your most attractive? Firming and toning your body can give you a glowing, youthful appearance, regardless of your age. The body that is strong and fit is also a healthier body. It will reduce your risk of developing many kinds of illnesses and diseases, make everyday life a joy, and can even add years to your lifespan. There is much more to a great body than simply looking good in a swimsuit!

Your goals should be sensible. While you may be able to obtain the body of a female bodybuilder, this is not a common goal for most women. You probably want to get the body you have in its best possible condition, so that you will feel and be more attractive. You probably also want the strong, toned body that reflects good health.

If these are your goals, physical fitness is your answer. You can choose the home workout routines which not only move you toward your goal, but are also much fun to do. Your home workout program will be much more satisfying, and you will be more likely to reach your goals, if you do not start with routines that are too physically-taxing or dull.

Starting with simple routines instead will give you two benefits. First, you will be less likely to incur injury; and second, when you choose fun routines, you will be more likely to continue them faithfully. Your workouts will be something to look forward to, each and every day.

Any woman can have a more attractive, healthier body. Most women can obtain amazing results. The key is to take your circumstances into consideration, and begin your workouts with enthusiasm. You can have that perfect body you have always wanted if you start slowly and proceed with consistency.

Special Situations

You are thinking about that perfect body. You may wonder if you have what it takes to obtain it. You may have a special situation which is leading you to doubt whether a home workout is for you. After all, the idea of starting a workout routine, and aiming for the body of your dreams, is quite new to you.

The good news is that home workouts are a great option for nearly anyone. Even if there is something different about your particular situation, you can turn it into something positive for working out.

One situation is the person who has neglected his body for many years. Not only has he become out-of-shape, flabby, and weak, the body that is not properly cared for often suffers in terms of health. You may be considerably overweight, even obese. If this sounds like you, you may be thinking that a home workout program would be useless, if not hazardous.

In this kind of situation, slowly-but-surely is the key to success. Beginning your workout program with easy exercises will help your body to become accustomed to its new adventure. While it is necessary to follow your physician's recommendations, it is not impossible for you to move in the direction of a healthy, fit body. In fact, it is simpler than you may believe.

The body that has been neglected will take more time to get into shape. This is only logical. However, you must not give up on yourself before you begin! You may be carrying more than a hundred extra pounds, and you may have fallen into the sedentary lifestyle of a couch-potato. With effort, hard work and determination, you can shed those extra pounds, and be physically fit and healthy again!

A second situation involves youngsters who are longing for that perfect body. It must be stressed that children and adolescents who are still growing should not take on a strenuous workout routine without their doctor's approval. This does not mean that working out is not suitable for children and teens. It only means that special attention must be focused on their growth stage.

When you keep this in mind, developing a good home workout program is one of the best things you can do for your child. He will learn to associate exercise with fun, and he will become stronger and healthier at the same time. When you provide your youngster with a workout program that is appropriate for his age and stage of physical development, you are teaching him good habits that will benefit him throughout his entire lifetime.

Many people who have physical impairments or disabilities also want to improve their bodies. It can give them more self-confidence, and be a boost to their overall health. If you have a disability or a medical condition which could interfere with the safety of a home workout program, it is advisable to check with your doctor before you begin. He can help you to customize a workout that is based on your special needs.

Some people have the idea that working out is only for young adults. They may believe that once a person reaches a certain age, working out is useless, and even dangerous. The good news is that nearly anyone who is reasonably healthy is not only capable of working out, but can benefit from a solid workout program.

You may be forty or sixty years of age, and not at all pleased with the condition of your body. You may be listening to friends or family members who tell you that you must accept this as a natural part of aging. This is not true at all! While your age may require you to impose sensible limitations on working out, you will be delighted with the results. You can have the fit, firm body that you recall from decades in the past, increase your overall health, and have a general sense of wellbeing. Working out at home can be the best decision you have ever made!

Almost anyone can benefit from working out. Most people can gain positive results. If you have any of these or other special situations, do not dismiss the idea of a home workout program. Regardless of your situation, a program can be custom-tailored, just for you. Your doctor and a physical fitness trainer can provide the advice you need to get on the right track.

As long as you proceed in a sensible manner, and keep your expectations reasonable, the odds are on your side that you will be successful. Home workouts are not only for the young, the person with unlimited time and resources, or the person who has athletics in mind. The benefits you gain from your workouts will have you convinced within a very short period of time. Anyone can look his best, and feel his best-- and this means you, regardless of your personal situation.

Forming that Muscle

When you think of a perfect body, what is the first thing to come to mind? You may be thinking of how great you will look in a new swimsuit, on the beach. You may be thinking about how much better you will look in your everyday clothes, when your body is in ideal condition.

Building muscle is the key to that perfect body. Whether you are naturally thin, or whether you are overweight and out of shape, it is muscle that will give your body the look you want.

This is why exercise routines which focus on building muscle are the foundation to a good home workout program. While increasing your body's overall strength, building solid muscle mass will firm and tone your contours. From biceps to abs to thighs, solid muscle will change your acceptable body into your ideal body.

If you are currently overweight, taking off pounds should not be your main focus. Instead, your workout program should reflect the process of turning unsightly fat into strong, healthy muscle. When your body starts to become firm, you will notice the difference. While solid muscles have weight, it is much different from the fat which you have been carrying! Toned muscles will give your body the shape you want, so that you will look better than ever before.

If you are naturally slim, you may be bothered by your thinness as much as the person who is overweight. Building muscle will give your body the bulk it needs to be stronger and more attractive. After you begin your new home workout program, you may be surprised at how quickly you start to see results. When you adhere faithfully to your workout program, your mirror will be all that you need to notice your hard work paying off.

Building muscle from working out is as appropriate for women as it is for men. While this is true for women in general, it is especially beneficial for women who are in their childbearing years. In addition to all of the other benefits, building strong, solid muscle can make pregnancy and childbirth much easier.

Pregnancy and childbirth place a considerable amount of stress on the body. Logically, the better shape your body is in, the better it is prepared for these processes. Strong muscles are what your body needs to work at its best. When your body is well-prepared with strong muscles, not only will your months of pregnancy be much smoother and more comfortable, it can contribute to an easier childbirth. It will help natural delivery to proceed faster, less painfully, and with a lower risk of complications.

Children and older persons benefit from building muscle, also. The youngster who has begun to build solid muscle from home workouts will find his natural growth spurts to be less troublesome. When coupled with a healthy lifestyle, it will also reduce his risk of becoming obese.

Older persons who build muscle will also benefit. The older person who is physically fit, with strong muscles, is less susceptible to falls and other accidents which are common amongst elderly people who are weak and out of shape. It will give him better mobility, and add to his overall quality of life. He will feel better about himself, and enjoy his life much more in his golden years.

When you first started thinking about that perfect body, your first emphasis was probably on appearance. After all, it is only natural to want to look your very best. You want to feel good about the way you look, and possibly even impress others! As you have been reading through this book, you have noticed more, equally important factors. You have learned that developing your ideal body is much, much more than having a body you will want to show off in a swimsuit. You have learned that a strong, physically-fit body is the number-one key to a healthier life.

Fortunately, the old saying "You cannot have it all" is not true. You can have physical fitness, glowing health, and the impressive body that you have always wanted. There is no miracle that can give you all of this. You must be willing to put the time and work into it. When your muscles start to become firmer and solid, you will notice the difference in your appearance. You will also feel the difference. The newfound strength in your body will be astonishing. Building muscle may feel as if you have been given a new lease on life, regardless of your age or physical condition.

You really can have it all-- and when you focus on building muscle with your home workout program, you will soon start to see the proof!

Chapter 4- Stay Focussed

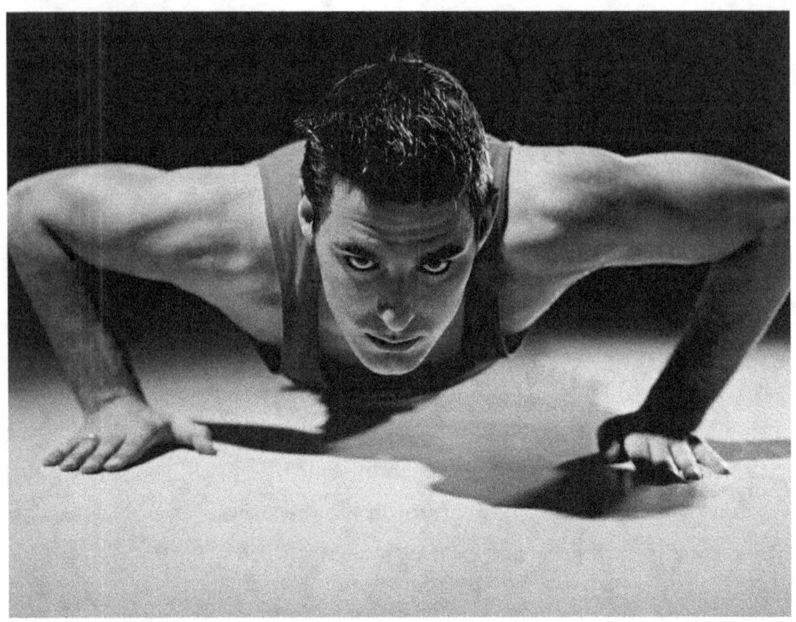

Some people sabotage their goals before they even begin. If you want success with your home workout program, you cannot afford to have this happen to you. Some tips to help you to be goal-oriented may be exactly what you need to transform your workout program into an exciting, successful experience.

There are two common mistakes which are often made in home workout programs. One mistake is to focus on your ultimate goal, and nothing else. If you use this method, you may soon begin to feel overwhelmed, overburdened, and frustrated. After all, nothing worthwhile was ever accomplished overnight.

Rather than making this mistake, you should consider the entire process. Instead of looking at your ultimate goal, you should appreciate every step you take to get there. Each day's workout is a success in itself, as it takes you that much closer to your goal.

You can set smaller goals along the way, and reward yourself for each one you attain. With this method, you are not only moving closer to that perfect body, you are also enjoying and appreciating all of the effort you are putting into it. This will help you to look forward to each workout, and see each one as progress.

The other common mistake is to overdo the focus on individual workouts, thinking that each one should provide miraculous results. If you find yourself stepping on the scale or reaching for a measuring tape after every workout, you are likely to become frustrated and disappointed very quickly.

Being sensible about what you can expect from your workouts can solve this problem. If you view each workout as one step on the ladder, you will find them much more satisfying. It is a positive way to appreciate your hard work.

One idea is to keep a diary of your workout program. Jotting down a brief note after every workout can help you to keep track of what you are doing. It will give you a basic framework of how much you are accomplishing, and how much more you still need to do. It is also something nice to look back on once you have reached your goals. When you notice how much effort you have put into your workouts, you will appreciate your success even more!

When you first decided to try a home workout program, you may have had a different method of being goal-oriented. Perhaps you had seen someone on television, and admired how great the person looked. Perhaps you saw a picture in a magazine, and wished that you could look so amazing. When you are goal-oriented, it does not need to be merely wishful thinking! You can have a prefect body, just like those people you see in the media. All you have to do is know where you are, where you want to go, and how to arrive.

There is a little something extra to this aspect of being goal-oriented. If the person you admire the most is clearly showing his natural body, without any photographic enhancements or anything else unnatural, this can be a very good way to become more goal-oriented. Instead of envying the person with the perfect body, you can remind yourself that he had to work to get to where he is. He was not born with handsome muscles and a lean physique-- he had to work hard for many months, possibly years, to look this way!

Reminding yourself that anything good takes time, hard work, and a great deal of patience, is the right way to become and to stay goal-oriented. While it may sound odd, or even a bit childish, posting a picture of someone with that perfect body where you can see it on a regular basis can be more useful than you realize. You can also tape or glue it onto the cover of your workout diary. It can provide that little extra bit of motivation, just when you need it the most!

Being goal-oriented does not mean focusing on your goal. Emphasizing the results you want can be counter-productive if it is not accompanied by the process. Like the old saying "Rome was not built in a day," the perfect body was not achieved overnight. No one can gain all of the results they desire from one or two workout sessions. It requires the commitment of being both oriented to your goal, and appreciative of everything you need to do to get there, for you to have that body of your dreams.

It can take a long time to reach your goal of a perfect body. When you think of it in terms of redesigning your entire body, changing everything that has been adequate or neglected thus far into something spectacular, you cannot afford to be in too much of a hurry. After all, whatever your current age may be, you have gone this far in your lifetime without the workouts your body requires to be in top-notch condition.

A year, or perhaps more, is not too much to expect. When you do not demand overnight results, you will see results much sooner. Every small success, when it is acknowledged and appreciated, brings you that much closer to your ultimate goal.

Diet and Supplements

You are almost ready to start the wonderful adventure of home workouts! You have your goals in mind, and are willing to work toward them. You are making your plan for exercising, equipment you want to buy, and scheduling time into your day to put it all into practice. You are motivated, enthusiastic, and prepared! There is a little more which you must do before you begin.

When you are looking forward to that perfect body, strength, vigor, and all-around health are as important as your exciting new appearance. As you have already learned in this book, when home workouts are done on a regular basis, it can be one of the most positive factors in good health and a longer lifespan. However, if you want the very best results, some changes to your lifestyle are also necessary.

One lifestyle change involves your diet. Whether your diet has been relatively good, or whether you have spent years surviving on junk-food, planning your home workout program is the perfect time to implement some changes.

A healthy diet does not require a professional dietician's input. All you really need to do is make a point of purchasing and eating healthy foods, and eliminating foods that are high in empty calories. If you want the perfect body, now is the time to give up carbonated soft drinks, alcohol, and other products which may taste good but do nothing for your body.

Fitness is Sexy

A healthy diet will make you healthier, of course. It also provides another benefit. Foods that are high in protein, and those that are rich in carbohydrates, provide long-lasting energy. When your diet contains plenty of these foods, not only will your workouts be easier, but your entire day will fill with natural energy.

Sweet foods and snacks give the opposite effect. They will cause your blood-sugar level to rise abruptly, and allow you to feel more energetic for a short period of time. As the effects of the sugar do not last long, your energy level will drop lower than it was before. Keeping your use of sugary snacks to a minimum will allow your energy level to remain consistent.

Dietary changes for the perfect body should include plenty of fruits, vegetables, and grain products. You will be amazed at how great you feel when these kinds of foods are the main focus of your daily diet. Equally important, the nutrients they provide will make you healthier than you ever were before. Your body's systems will work better, and you will feel great!

When you are beginning a new home workout program, do not underestimate your body's need for fluid. While this is important in general, it is even more relevant when you are doing strenuous exercise. Fresh water, cool fruit drinks, and drinks which are specially made for this purpose, will keep your body hydrated. Sports drinks which are designed to replace and balance electrolytes are a good choice.

Exercise depletes the body's natural fluids. It often happens quite rapidly. Losing fluid through perspiration can make you feel run-down and tired, as well as undermining your body's overall health. Be sure that you have plenty of liquid on hand to drink during your workout, and to drink afterward. It is essential to replenish your body's natural fluids.

Planning your home workout program to include lifestyle changes should also include the use of supplements. No matter how healthy your diet may be, the lack of any essential nutrients can impede your progress. For example, you might not be aware of how minerals can be lost through normal perspiration. This is especially true when you are perspiring excessively during workouts.

Multi-vitamin and mineral supplements are a positive addition to your home workout program. You do not have to spend a fortune on name-brand supplements. With a little comparison-shopping, you can less expensive supplements that provide all of the nutritional elements you need. Choosing a good multi-vitamin and mineral supplement for your daily use is more than a good decision to add to your workout program-- it is a healthy habit that will benefit you for the rest of your life.

You may be wondering why a home workout program contains so many more extras than you had initially considered. The reason for this is that a perfect body requires much more than some basic exercises and equipment. If you want your workout program to be truly productive, you must focus on your entire body as a whole. This means getting healthier, increasing your stamina, and making sure that your body has everything it needs for a rigorous workout and all the years ahead.

As you have learned in this book, there is much to do, and much to gain from doing it. At times, it may not be easy, but it is not complicated. When you know what you want, and are willing to do the work to achieve it, that perfect body can be yours!

Success!

If you have been approaching the subject of home workouts with the goal of a perfect body in mind, there is one additional point to consider. While you may have much to overcome in order to get the great body you are dreaming of, you cannot allow success to mean complacency. What we mean by this is that even after you reach your goal, you can backslide if you do not continue the practices and habits you have learned in this book.

When you reach success, you have so many reasons to be proud of yourself! It takes work, motivation, time, commitment, and determination to gain that perfect body! When you reach your goal, you surely do not want to risk losing it.

Instead of looking at your home workout program as a means to an end, think of it as habits and practices that will benefit you throughout the rest of your lifetime. While you may not need to continue the same exercise routines as you use to get into shape, you must continue exercising to stay in shape. Otherwise, the solid muscle you have put so much time into building and perfecting can lose its tone.

The same is true with your dietary changes. When you get into the habit of eating only nutritious foods, and taking dietary supplements, you must look forward to continuing this practice for the rest of your life.

While a little backsliding is natural, you do not want to risk everything which you have worked so hard to attain. Making your program a lifetime program will help to ensure that you keep it. You can look great, feel great, and even proceed into old age when you make it all a part of your everyday life.

The success of a perfect body does not come easily, or quickly. Now that you know the steps you need to take to reach your goal, it can happen for you! You will surely be delighted with the results!

Chapter 5- Listen To The Expert Before Getting Fit

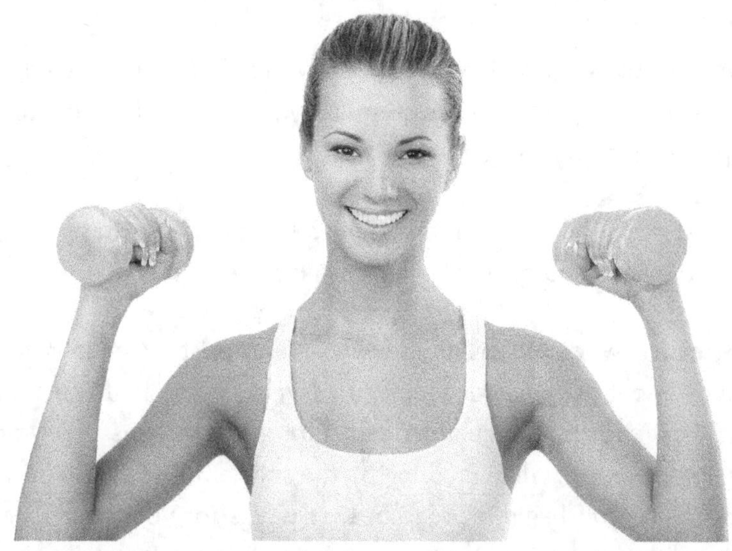

Working out is imperative to avert particular illnesses, such as high cholesterol, high- blood pressure, diabetes, heart failure, and strokes. Exercise can also reduce your risks of encountering cancerous illnesses. Furthermore, exercise will strengthen the bones and muscles, which decreases your chances of fallen susceptible to fractures, breaks, back injuries and/or diseases and so on.

Eating unhealthy provisions is not an answer for promoting good health. Some people exercise yet eat fast foods, which only defies the purpose of promoting good health. The body will not respond friendly when unhealthy foods and exercise work against each other.

Rest is also important, since if you are not getting proper rest, while exercising you are subjecting self to fainting, hot flashes, and other negative results. The body responds to motion or active forces while exercising, thus during the process the body expects vigilance to function without complexity. If the body is tired, the body and mind will respond accordingly which could lead to passing out and injuring self as a result.

Working out is an active force that works to produce healthier lives, while reducing the risks of ordinary disease, at the same time helping you to control your weight?

At what time you work out and have a basic idea of what you are doing the body and mind will make available good results.

Progressive work out plans may include consistent actions that include repetitions, cadenced, or rhythmic dance, bodily actions that work the total circulatory structure and exercises that work the large muscles, while focusing on the smaller muscles within the body. Once you begin a program that works for you, your blood flow will boost, which slowly expands to the muscles, supporting the cardiovascular strength.

Aerobics then is one of the finest exercise plans that can lend a hand to progressing toward a healthier living. Aerobics is a vigorous work out that works each muscle in the body, toning the body while increasing weight loss concurrently.

Aerobics include walking, running in place, jogging, swimming, skating, bicycling, dance as well as other types of aerobic exercise motions. Aerobics that comprise working the total body to build muscle, while it employs the larger muscles, and endorsing your cardiovascular strength are idea aerobics that will help you lose weight while staying healthy. If you merge aerobics with weight lifting you will be building muscles, mass, strengthening the bones, and reducing weight. You will reach a level of tone, firmness, and healthier status of living while combing the exercises.

Weight lifting is a shape of workouts that is alleged to lend a hand to individual's attempting to lose weight quickly, while building muscles. If your goal is to build muscle, you should be attentive that insubstantial weight lifting is almost certainly your best decision

Intense weight lifting is usually for weight lifters attempting to build mass muscles, such as body builders. If you do not want to resemble one of the body builders, then it is significant to learn the type of weight lifting program that is appropriate for you. Most information accessible brings up to date individuals, interested in weight lifting, telling them a variety of methods (all with diverse notions) which plan is right for them; it is vital then that you keep the routines in moderation while starting out, regardless of the advice you receive. Typically, thirty minutes in weight lifting per day or every 3 days is adequate for building muscle and toning the body. Over and above this advice while heavy weight lifting may result in mass muscle, build.

If you ignore this advice, do not blame me when you start to look like Hulk Hogan. While training myself, I found that working out three times per week during the morning time worked best, but my body type differs from yours so find what works best for you.

Building muscles by working out you should first learn which exercises are paramount to your body type. It is wise to stick with a diet that works best for you also. Do not forget to rest and drink plenty of water.

Experts are continually learning innovative particulars regarding the body, nevertheless, the information accessible concerning body types is a foundation to relating to the type of body, which assists in determining which diet plans work paramount to your body type.

When consider body type one should stay alert to the types of exercises that suit the body type best. The hormones are essential when considering exercises. The hormones are chemical dispatch riders, which send communiqué to the electrical system within the body. The electrical system is also known as the Central Nervous System (CNS), which includes the brainpower.

The hormones decide on the person's thoughts, feelings, and how a person will develop according to the experts. The body composes cells, nerve endings, nuclei, which are a cluster of chemicals produced in brain cells, glands, and various other organs, which influence a huge number of functionalities within the body.

Hormones producing such chemicals only drop or raise the aging process. The hormones will determine the amount of pain and anguish our health will endure, as well as affecting the metabolism, while deciding on the body's mass, or weight. The hormones indirectly or directly affect the person's height, perception, memory, blood pressure, digestion system, just to name a few. Hormones send chemicals to the endocrines gland, which the consequences is the secreting of hormone dispatching in to the bloodstream. The affect is that the body's functional system of cells and other organ's affect the entire body. Thus, the CNS also plays a large role in the changes our body accepts.

As you can see, the body requires balance. Balance is part of losing weight. The Endomorph then is a body type that often has large bones, huge trunk area, spherical face, and thighs, which has a lot of body fat biologically. The body fat on this type is often found near the midsection, which means these types of body's fight back to preserve weight or else lose weight.

The Endomorph body type demands motivations higher than the MESOMORPH AND ECTOMORPH types. This is necessary to maintain weight. Thus, burning fat, increasing metabolism, and including low-intense exercises combined with high-endurance exercises is the idea combo for this type of body, yet devoid of over training.

Endomorph bodies tend to work best at the lesser objective heart rate precinct. The body requires oxygen, which must flow smoothly to increase your health and reduce the weight, or maintain a weight level.

Once the body develops or adjusts, you will need to increase the volume of exercises. The endomorph types are told to reduce the caloric intakes, while consuming an abundance of low caloric provisions.

MESOMORPH types are more of the bodybuilding types. The MESOMORPH body can enjoy high-intense weight lifting with ease, while enjoying temperate aerobics.

The MESOMORPH body has larger bones and thicker skin, thus dieting should include low-fat provisional foods, with advanced caloric intake. The MESOMORPH body often pans out as the body decreases fat intake and increases calorie intakes, providing the person conform to regular workout schemes.

The ECTOMORPH type has lower body fat, with high volumes of mass. These types are said to suffer repeated hot flashes, since the fat in the body is lacking. The

ECTOMORPH types require more fatty foods to maintain a level of weight, and an extreme intake of calories than other types.

The ECTOMORPH has difficulty gaining weight, thus the body requires heavy weight lifts with increasing repetitions after the body adjusts. The hormones playing a large role, brings us to the point. Regardless of the body type, we all have hormones, which mean we need a balanced diet and proper exercises to promote hormonal producing, endomorph producing, and other productions that the body demands.

With this in mind you also want to consider Glycogen and Oxygen, which both play a major part in weight gain or lose. While experts all have their idea as to what keys in to good health and fitness, it is up to us to find what works best for our body. Cross training is said to be one of the better solutions for burning fat, reducing calories, losing weight, building strength and so on.

More Advice

According to few insulin levels play the largest role in losing weight. Other experts determine that our body type is the key to finding the proper exercises and diet plans that work with the body.

To achieve a healthier status and maintain weight diet must combine with exercise, since one without the other will not work. Combining healthy provisions with correct exercises can bring you good health and physical fitness, which will enhance your quality of life. It will also help you keep your body's zone to a level.

The body and mind is complicated, however both work together to produce results. Many experts, including theorists, doctors, scientist, and philosophers are continuing to find answers to the body's functions.

Some of the confusion comes when people diet, exercise and take care of them self, yet they still gain weight. Barry Sears wrote a compelling book titled A Week in the Zone, which produced some outstanding advice. Some of the information in the book helps us to decide on exercises and diets that suit us best, since insulin plays a large part in healthier living.

The author lets us know that the hormones consequence of intakes of carbohydrates and caloric differ from the hormones that produce protein and calories. , he continues letting us know that the effects of hormones that produce fats and calories too differ in the direction of health. (p. 3)

The author brings us to see that a balance is needed, yet the balance is factored by the different hormonal levels. Thus, eating healthy, giving the body proper fluids and exercising is the only answer to living a productive and quality lifestyle.

One of the biggest setbacks that people adhere to is making excuses to avoid dieting and exercise. Countless of people find it easier said than done to stick with diet and exercise programs that facilitates them to remain healthy while maintaining weight.

One of the largest reasons is that most people do not understand their body and its type, or have difficulty adhering to a schedule. One of the largest reasons why this happens is that many people find it difficult to plan, set goals that work, and find solutions that help the person maintain a schedule. The threesome is the ultimate tools for working toward good health and fitness.

If you are uncertain of the types of exercises, this too can hold you back. Walking up and down the stairs is an aerobic exercise. Mowing the lawn is another type of exercise. Anytime the body is in motion, producing actions it is exercising. Lifting 12' ounces of beer is not an exercise. Alcohol if overused will affect the body and mind dramatically.

Other forms of exercise are merely walking to the store instead of driving your car, especially if the store is down the road. If you find it, difficult getting started with exercise makes effort to ask a friend or family member to join you. Otherwise, possibly at your workplace a team of people is joining a gym to better their health, maybe you can go with them. If you have a dog, dogs enjoy walking, therefore put your feet in motion and make your dog happy. Children also enjoy walking with parents, therefore spend time with your children and exercise while doing so.

Therefore, if you have intricacy with setting goals, planning, or sticking to a schedule, begin by using the stairs in place of an elevator at what time you visit your doctor, or other appointments. In addition, you could scythe the lawn in place of paying the fellow citizen down the street to do the work for you. Beginning exercise is by no means easy, but you have to start somewhere to reach a healthier status!

The Body's Zone

What would you say if someone told you in seven days you could live a healthier lifestyle, while feeling better and working to live longer? This is one of the repeated ad slicks that tell you in a short time you can lose weight in a single week. If you are taking pills this is not going to happen, however if you are exercising and abiding by a diet you may lose a pound or two in a week.

New studies show that if you continue insulin degree, meaning that if the insulin is neither low nor high, your probability of living a healthier life increases. The Zone is essential for maintaining physical fitness and living a healthier life. The Zone processes chemicals in the body, which fight heart disease. However, exercise and healthy provisions are needed to divert diabetes and other diseases as well as burning fat, while keeping the insulin level. The insulin level will help fight cancer, as well as other diseases and will prevent depression. Thus, to keep fit then, the body's zone must maintain a level of insulin that is neither low nor high.

At what time the body's zone is high or low, the health starts to deteriorate. To uphold our health we must learn a variety of details pertaining to the body's internal productions. Insulin is merely a hormone in the body, which is hidden by the cells. Hormones comprise protein. This means that insulin is also protein. At what time the body digest provisions that enclose Carbohydrates, the body's insulin secretes. The secretion is by the pancreas, which passes onto the intestines, thus extending through the bloodstream. This process determines the level of the blood pressure. Sugars in Carbohydrates engross foremost into the intestines, which ultimately arrives at the bloodstream, thus insulin at this point begins its work.

At what time the insulin level becomes either low or high, the zone is affected in more than a few ways. If the insulin maintains a level, thus it can help the body improve its performance while preventing various diseases, including diabetes. According to Barry Sears (PhD), the author of A Week in the Zone at what time a person maintains insulin, the body begins utilizing fats, using them as vigor, which permits lose of disproportionate body fats devoid of experiencing the feeling of famine. (p. 1)

Still, we need exercise to maintain a healthy life. If the body zone is healthier, it is even better to start exercising now. If you are not working out, the zone will overtime drop below health endurance. Barry lets us know that if the level of insulin is normal, we have better odds of enjoying a longer lifespan, while maintaining mental awareness. Thus, the insulin level determines our fitness and health. One of the reasons that people endure obesity according to Barry is that overwhelming amounts of hormonal insulin controls the body. Barry states that insulin is what makes the body gain weight and holds the weight. (p. 2-3)

Exercise is THE primary factor that helps us to maintain good health. At what time the body is in motion and stretching on a daily basis, the body responds accordingly by providing flexibility and ease of movement. Thus, the motion enables the insulin and bloodstream to flow at a normal rate.

Even if the health is poor, or the person has diabetes, the primary advice your doctor will give you is to walk a mile daily. When a person walks, it works the cells, nerves, circulation, muscles, and the whole body in general. Thus, the chief goal then to promoting health and fitness is maintaining a normal insulin level, while keeping the body fit by adhering to exercises and diet.

Barry also makes a point in his book that calories and intake of fat is misconstrued. Barry tells us that 'fat' houses 'more calories' per each gram of fat, than carbohydrates and protein contain. This brings us to believe that reducing fat can make a person slimmer. Barry claims that the level of hormones is also equilibrium. The body requires a degree of fat, carbohydrates, caloric intake, and protein to work productively. Therefore, the diet that is right for you decide on your body type, insulin level, and other factors.

CHAPTER 6- AEROBICS FOR FITNESS

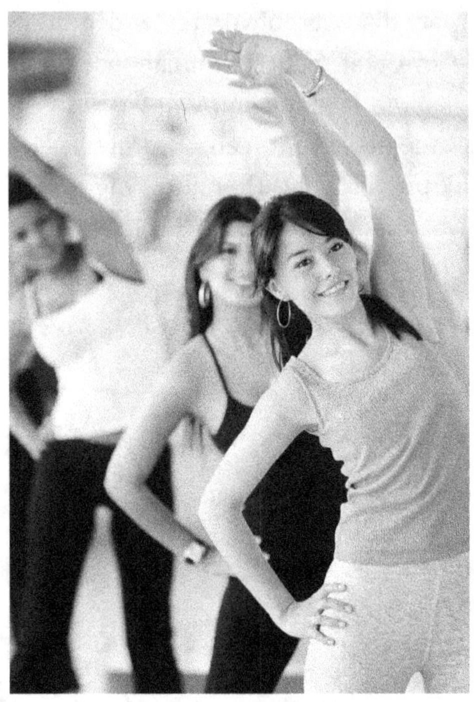

Since Health and Fitness Gyms opened novel aerobic exercises came into play. At the gyms around the world, you can join in Cardio Kick Boxing, Hip Hop Aerobics, Striptease and Martial Arts Aerobics and so on.

Cardio Kick Boxing is comparable to Martial Arts Aerobics, in that it comprises karate into a workout routine... Some of the Martial Arts Aerobics comprise Kick Skills, Choreography, Warm-ups, punches, and so on with each working the complete body.

Striptease Aerobic depend on the trainer, but in few Aerobic Striptease workouts the routine comprises basic spinning, pole dances, transitional and progressive spins, and advanced turn upside down moves. The dance moves could comprise advanced to beginner steps. If you want to become an exotic dancer, this is the aerobics of choice. In fact, this particular aerobics routine was shown on the Oprah Winfrey show. It was brought out in the show that this particular aerobics brings out sexual appeal while toning the body.

If you cannot afford to visit the Gyms, you may want to consider learning home aerobics. The exercises can benefit you, while you work out in the comforts of your home. Few of the fundamental aerobics comprise using the Nordic Track Skier, climbing stairs, jogging around the room, walking in repetition, bicycling, running, canoeing, or using a Video that composes all the steps you need to acquire fitness and health. Most of the aerobics will work the bulky muscles metrically and incessantly, while elevating the hearts rate. Other exercises including racquetball, tennis, dance, and roller blade and or skating can also enhance your health while you work toward fitness. It is important to check with your physician before starting any aerobic routines and/or other types of exercises.

Nearly everyone running Aerobic classes begin the routines with warm-ups and stretches, while progressively working into a temperate workout. Few instructors will increase velocity following temperate training completion, but few trainers may not. Few trainers are already in to their own routine and fail to see that beginners join their classes. Still, it depends on the instructor. The process of aerobics is intended to amplify the rate of the heart, boost awareness of the body, elevating the body's temperature, and increasing the flow of blood, extending to the muscles.

Aerobics are superior for increasing the heart rate, for restoring the cardio respiratory staying power, while utilizing the larger muscles. Aerobics also enhances the body's composition.

Once you complete a full exercise routine, you will move toward a cool-down workout. It is important to stretch and do warm-ups before aerobics or exercises, as well as cooling down after you finish a routine. The cool-down is intended to reduce the rate of the heartbeats, while averting extreme pooling the blood in the lesser farthest point. Thus, any aerobic routine should include stretches and relaxing workout at the start and completion. The routine helps to shun soreness in the muscles, while enhancing flexibility, and reinstating the balance and/or homeostasis. Furthermore, the cool-down will help to decrease the rate of which the heart beats.

The Hip-hop Aerobics is a boogie aerobic, which combines modern dance with funk. Hip-Hop Aerobics comprises steps that increase energy, while focusing on the entire form of the body. The workout is outstanding for beginners. If you never danced before, perk up those engines because now you will learn to move and groove while working toward fitness and health. If you are trying to lose weight fast, this is the idea aerobics of choice.

The Hi-Lo Aerobic routines work the thighs, heart, abs, calf and so on. Beginners are wise to choice the Hip-Hop or other type of aerobics and work toward this exercise, since it involves rapid movements. The individual moves frequently on one side while slanting in position. The Hi-Lo involves shuffling, turning, shuffling some more, and doubling the knees back while sprinting during the routine and then taking a deep side lunge at speedy pace.

Funk and Jazz Aerobics comprise low-impacting workouts, which generally include jazz steps, funk twists and yoga. Some include the PILATE aerobics, but mostly the exercise is great for newcomers into the gym, since no heavy gear is involved. The routine is generally temperate.

Boogie Aerobics

Aerobic dances have been fashionable in the past few years. In the precedent decades, fitness and health centers have grown, extending on their routines and weight ideas offered. Most health and fitness clubs present an assortment of exercises, including weight lifts, PILATES, yoga, aerobics, spinning, kick boxing, karate, and more.

The selection of health and fitness clubs frequently have their own exclusive styles to assist individual's in losing weight, increasing muscle mass, toning the bodies, strengthen the bones and so on. Aerobic exercises have tempting headings intended to catch the eye. The titles include the Hi-Lo aerobics, Aerobics rooted on Martial Arts, Aerobic Striptease, Cardio Kick Boxing, Hip-Hop, Funk and Jazz, and so on. Some of the aerobic routines include equipment to enhance exercise and fitness experiences.

Slide or Step Aerobics implicates equipment. During the Step Aerobics routines, you position a footstep in the frontage, which you step one foot up, down and up on the other leg, replicating the course of action for quite a few minutes. The process is intended to tone the lower body; still concerns of Step Aerobics have made statements, since the ankles and knees are normally utilized often.

The Slide Aerobics involves a step, and in its place of stepping up repetitiously to the frontage, the work outer steps to the side, slide downward, and then slides back up. The Slide Aerobics show a discrepancy in each Health and Fitness Gyms. Some Slide Aerobics might implicate equipment, including the Nordics Ski.

Before joining a Health and Fitness Club, make sure you are aware of the types of aerobics offered to you, since few clubs might offer more affective aerobic courses than others will. Some clubs have trainers available willing to help you choose the right aerobics for you, while other clubs merely want their pay. For example, some clubs may offer aerobic routines that focus on flexibility. The aerobic routines will mostly involve stretches, which means you will not receive the results you are possibly searching to achieve, including losing weight fast.

Hi-Lo Aerobics flowing

Hi-Lo Aerobics involves a fast-paced routine that includes rapid movement. The individual moves typically on the side and in a slanting position. During the Hi-Lo you will shuffle, turn, shuffle, and double the knee back, while sprinting during, and taking a profound side lunge at swift paces. The Hi-Lo aerobics work the Calf, Thighs, Abs, Heart Legs, and so on. Beginners would benefit more by choosing a different type of aerobics exercise, since the Hi-Lo is more for the advanced. The main idea of aerobics is not hurting your self-while better your health.

Hip-hop Aerobics is a dance routine, which mix together funk with contemporary dance. The Aerobic dance implicates the usage of high-energy dance, while working out the complete body. The work out is optional, but works for everyone. If you are a novice who knows nothing about dancing, do not fret, as the instructor will direct you through the process; include teaching you the grooves, rhythm, rhyme and moves. If you are training to lose weight, the Hip-Hop is a first-class alternative to decide on, since dance has proven to be one of the most effective exercises to date.

Funk and Jazz aerobics depend on the Fitness and Health Center, as to what the Aerobics include, but few clubs merge low-impact work out that often includes exhilarating jazz dances with a twist of funk and yoga. Funk and Jazz is an option for beginners, since the training does not include weighty equipment and the routines are temperate.

Cardio Kick Boxing relies on the trainer, but mainly Cardio Kick Boxing is an elevated work out for getting in shape promptly, while learning techniques to perk up physical robustness. The work out includes footwork while merging karate kicks and strikes. Cardio helps you to lose weight, tone the body, increase muscle, while teaching self- defense. Cardio Kick Boxing frequently comprises jump rope, crunches, stretches, bag punches, kicks, and pushups.

Dance Aerobics for the Beginners

Dance aerobics include steps, funk, and powering the rump. Persons that lack the artistic ability to dance may wonder why join a class that includes dancing. The trainers at most gyms have made it convenient for beginners to take the front in aerobic dance steps. The aerobics will tone the body, add volume, increase flexibility, and enforce staying power.

While you might find it difficult to learn that steps to perfection at first, in time, you will learn, but in the meantime, you are burning off those calories. When the body sweats because of movement, the calories start to burn, which in turns reduces pounds.

After joining a class, you will quickly learn why continuing dance aerobics is smart. The dance aerobics is the better option for increasing the hearts muscle, while increasing oxygen levels at the same time. Dance aerobics enhance metabolism, while improving balance.

After getting started, your body will take you, since it will feel great. Aerobics that include dance steps may entail stepping forward on one foot, while raising the knees simultaneously on the other leg. One other well-known step in aerobics that includes dance steps is marching in place. Overall, it is vital that you learn minimal details pertaining to the exercise, including what gear to wear, which will include shoes and clothes.

Other steps in dance aerobics include spinning, twirling, and moving the feet in motion to the beat. Since dance aerobics not only involves dancing in place, it is important that you wear that appropriate attire and shoes. If you fail to adhere to advice, the dance aerobics might end up being an uncomfortable routine. Avoiding the right attire and shoes can also lead to injury.

The body sweats during any workout. Therefore, wearing fitting clothes is essential when dancing. Weightless clothes are the choice, since it helps while you sweat, and the right clothes can support breasts, especially for women. Jocks are recommended if men are joining dance aerobics.

While participating at your first dance class, it is wise to show up at least fifteen minutes early. Instructors are available during training, and if you show up early, the instructor can learn your status in the club. The instructor can spend a few minutes, to make sure you are spotted appropriately.

If you are a beginner, it is advised that you participate in dance aerobic classes that start with basic dance steps. The classes that employ the Hi-Lo dance moves are the best option for beginners. The step-funk and power the rump classes are more for the advanced trainers, thus if you cannot dance, this is not idea for you.

Dancing is an art, which requires mastering overtime. Some people require experience, while others learn rapidly. Few of the better dancers on Television start out as novice dancers, and few did not have a starting point. Once you get into the groove however, learning a few moves, it shouldn't take long to learn a few more steps. If you are not dance oriented, this too will become noticeable.

If large crowds make you, nervous you may want to pay attention at the mirrors located in the Gym. The mirrors are often attached to the walls, and surround the entire workout area. Consequently, if you are anxious at what time you walk in the entrance, it might be to your advantage to watch the mirrors and avoid looking at the trainers. Make certain that you keep an eye on the instructor so that you do not fail to spot steps. An alternative, is following this priceless tip and avoid putting too much forethought into what the trainer is saying. Instead, put more scrutiny into what the trainer is doing. This will facilitate in decreasing anxiety.

In time, you will learn the steps in dance aerobics if you apply self. Exercises, especially those that work with the cardiovascular system, muscles and bones are the best form of exercises available. Dance in my experience, is one of the better choices of exercises that helps keep the body tone, firm, while maintaining weight.

Aerobics Cross Training Basic

Aerobics involve using the large muscles incessantly while moving the body in rhythmically motion. The routines enhance beats of the heart and smoothest the breathing repetitions. Full body aerobic exercises might comprise the basics, including dance, walking in place, ski, bicycling, running in place and jogging. It is important to learn about the aerobics before starting routines to avoid injury.

The objective is important before starting aerobics. Once you know your objective, you will know what you want from the exercises. You should also consider the condition of your health, including genetics and history of disease in the family. Preceding injuries should also be considered before starting aerobics.

To get started, what is your objective? Is your goal to lose weight and/or burn fat? If you have a goal in mind and it is to burn fat and lose weight considering your goal, health and history can help you avoid injury during workout and harm to injuries from the past. Cross training then, is one of the better choices of aerobics to prevent injuries. Cross training is merely combining one aerobic routine with another routine, such as half weights and aerobics. Cross training will help you achieve equilibrium of training schedules.

Before considering cross training however, we must understand the different exercises. Few exercises include the low-temperate workouts, high-impact workouts, and so on. If you are intending to lose weight and burn fat, combining the low and high-impact aerobics together can give you faster results. For example, if you include low-temperate aerobics with high-impact aerobics you might walk, step, ski, dance, run, or play racquetball. The idea timeframe is three to five days each week and at least one hour each set.

The mixture reduces risk especially if you suffer from preceding or present injury, including hip injury, low back injury, ankle, or other related injuries. If you have existing injury the experts tell you to workout in moderation, this is why it is important to consult with your doctor before starting aerobic routines. Most likely, the doctor will tell you to avoid ski exercises if you had prior injuries.

Cardiovascular exercise are intended to make available complete body augmentation while strengthen the muscles and bones. Of course, this includes strengthening of the joints, while reducing fats and calories. The cardio workouts will help develop muscles and boost Cardiovascular. Working out can enhance the body's flexibility as well. As you can see the correct cross-training routines is essential. If you are considering high- impact workouts, such as running you may want to combine bicycling, stretches and weights at least once each week. The combo will strengthen the muscles, while enhancing the body.

If you considered jogging, then it can enhance the fitness, while improving cardio. Jogging includes using the large muscles; however, the problem is that it will not increase mass also. Cross-training then will include working the upper body, which may include weights, or correct aerobics that work the upper body. In spite of everything, you are not acquiring flexibility, which the body demands. To include cross training exercises for flexibility, include stretching and warm-ups into your routine.

Experts of sport have claimed that cross training is one of the better choices, since it provides constructive results. Combing exercises is the hit of the higher points in physical working out.

Summing it up, cross-training exercises if choosing the correct combination, will burn fat, strengthen muscles and bones, reduce calories, and produce flexibility, while working the complete body. Cross training can lend a hand to individuals trying to build up the body. Cross training can also make available sources of pleasure, as well as enhancing energy levels, which includes building Metabolism.

If your goal is to acquire fitness, then you are required to comprise strength walking, vigorous walking, swim, jog, ski, bicycle riding, skating and other types of exercises into your routine. To strengthen the muscles use free weights, or isometric workouts. Isometric workouts are opposite muscle workouts that contract since it includes minuscule restraints but boost in tone of muscle fibers. It is important to keep fit if you want good health, therefore learn the right cross training steps for you.

CHAPTER 7- MUSCLE BUILDING: INCREASE STRENGTH

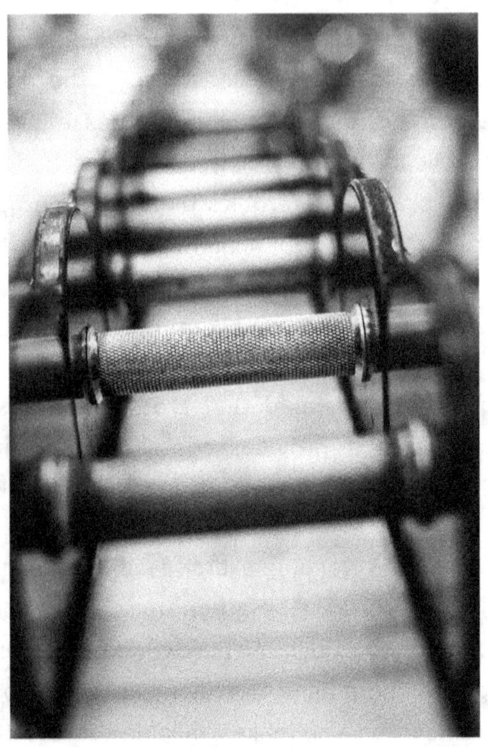

At what time you setup an exercising routine that includes aerobics, combing a routine composed of strength-building of muscles, the body is burning amino acids, fat, carbohydrates and protein.

At what time you exercise burning fats, Carbohydrates, and amino acid proteins, burning the body's requirements while in motion; you are losing weight, while building strength.

The body demands specific quantities of amino acids, fats and carbohydrates to function correctly. At what time you work out your body's glycogens and oxygen is working, (if the exercise routines are in temperance) as well the body is building form while tearing down the nutrients, which creates weight increase. Still the body's strength is decreasing.

Aerobics workouts not only manufacture oxygen, the workouts increase the cardiovascular arrangement. At the same time, the process restores oxygen, while increasing the heart muscles and its ability to work correctly. Thus, aerobics is a Strengthening of the heart, which promotes oxygen.

Having an overall understanding of Glycogen can facilitate why we should be grateful for the worth of aerobic oxygen. Glycogen distinctiveness is comprehended in more than a few areas. Glycogen either works with the body, or else in opposition of the body. In view of the fact that Glycogen is the leading element found in the muscle tissue and the liver, which liberally switches the glucose, which satisfies the vigor requirements of the body. At the same time, glycogen makes provisions for vigor, especially during intense workloads. The CNS or Central Nervous System relies on glycogen to increase vigor, thus if glycogen is low, our intensity of exercise is limited.

Thus, including weights and aerobics combing them to conform to a cross training scheme is idea for strength building. Working the muscles in groups can enhance our value of how Glycogen and Oxygen work together, yet help us to appreciate how much more significant Oxygen is to building strength over Glycogen.

Now you may wonder how strength is built, and how the body movements have an effect on the ability to strength build, but the answer is obvious. The proper exercises are necessary to build strength and this includes a plan or schedule where both aerobics and weights are included in the routine. The cross training scheme works to restore the muscles strength keeping the muscles in groups, and using oxygen and glycogen to do so.

Of course, you will need to consider the level of strength building you want to achieve, however moderate workouts can enhance your body in a short time. Intense-low weight lifting combined with temperate aerobics is idea of strength building, yet a well-balanced diet is also needed to restore the body's requirements once burnt.

Thus, in overall understanding when the muscles are not worked in groups, thus building strength is in process. Correct training can lend a hand by helping you stay bodily vigorous, while working toward fitness. As well, the correct training can make available a customary level for your body's function. Strength building is the procedure of moving the body on a recurring experience to preserve a degree of fitness and health. At what time the large muscles are in constant motion, working jointly with the smaller muscles, it provides unremitting corporeal fitness and health. The muscles expand as a person grows, as well as, the muscles modify as the years cultivates.

Thus, building strength broadens the muscles in the body, while endurance workouts increase formations of the blood vessels. The combo keeps the body strong and healthy, while declining the body's progression of aging. You can only go in the right directing by including correct training and diet into your living routines.

Our body is a stronghold. If we do not take care of our body, likely our body will let us down as the years grow. The mind also works to make the body produce either negative or positive results. Thus, the correct workouts and diets can also enhance the mind's ability to function properly. Even if you have a mental disability, exercise and diet can help you gain control of your life and health.

Stretches

Stretches is one of the most important exercises any of us can put into our daily schedule. The back especially requires stretches, since it is the producer of several body muscles. The back is often the first area where people experience pain. One of the first stretching exercises that target the back is the single exercise that will make the back release from pain. Other stretch exercises are important; however, the back requires added attention. During a day, we put a lot of weight on the back, since everything we do in a day's time, rely heavily on the back.

To start back exercises lay your back in a comfortable position with the legs elongated and the arms stretched over the head. It is vital that the back flex exercises are done correctly to avoid injury. With both hands stretched over the head stretch up as far as the arms will allow simultaneously stretching the legs at length. Make sure the chest is expanded up and hold your place up to fifteen or thirty seconds. Repeat until you feel the body release stress and tension.

The triceps stretches require bending the 'right arm' bending it behind the neck area. Bend the elbows extending them toward the ceiling. With the left hand clutching the right elbow, tug gently to the left until you feel a stretching sensation; At this point you should feel a stretching sensation at the rear of the higher right arm. Repeat the procedure on each arm holding in place both arms up to fifteen to thirty seconds.

The hip flexor stretch requires lunging to the front on one leg, while reaching the shoulders' at breadth, and steadying the feet on the floor. With your knee (right), rest the feet and toes on the floor in firm place. The knee (left) should be higher than the ankle. Lower the hip (right) steadily until a stretch feeling exists. Again, repeat fifteen to thirty seconds per leg.

Hamstrings require sitting in a relaxed position while bending the left leg, and extending the right. The left foot should be in a resting position while touching the inner portion of the other leg. (Right) Coil the higher portion of the body directing to the knee until it touches. A stretching feeling should exist around the right area of the hamstring. Hold position up to fifteen to thirty seconds and swap legs following the same procedure.

When doing calf stretches, you should stand in a comfortable position placing the "hands on the hip region. Calf Stretches can also be done by placing 'both hands on a wall (shoulder's width apart). Once you have positioned yourself, you will then step frontward 'with your right foot (about a half-shoulder's width). Then you will bend the knees, with your feet grounded to the floor, and shift your body 'to your forward foot." Once you have followed these procedures then you will lower your hips gradually, until your body exposes a mild stretching feeling in your "calf muscle and Achilles tendon." (Rear-left leg) Continue this for at least "15 to 30 seconds," on each leg.

Shoulder Stretches I recommend that a person does shoulder stretches first; however, each trainer has his/her own purposes and reasons why other stretches should be done first. To do proper shoulder stretches you will need to stand in a comfortable position, binding "your fingers behind your back so that your palms are facing in toward your spine, thumb" aiming toward the floor. Once you have positioned yourself properly, then proceed by linking your hands in the direction of the ceiling gradually, while your back and neck is in a relaxed state.

You should feel a stretching awareness in your chest. Continue the shoulder exercises for by holding in position "for 15 to 30 seconds. Neck Stretches Sitting flat on the floor, tilt your head in a backwards position. Tilt you head, rolling it from side to side.

Slightly lower your head toward your chest, moving it from side to side, and then to the back. Do not drop your head lower than needed to feel the stretch sensation that is most effective. After you have finished the flexibility exercises, you can then move on to a full body workout.

However once you have finished your workout, it is recommended that you do a cool down exercise, coupled with stretches. This will help your body to relax after you have endured a full body workout. Light flexibility exercises are great for limbering the body, and should be done before exercise begins to give your body the flexibility it needs to exert itself.

Stretching the Joints

It is important that our joints are strong and healthy to avoid arthritis. Other types of exercises are great for the body, which include exercises that strengthen bones, muscles and joints. It is important to consider all aspects of the body when exercising to get the best results of health and fitness.

Stair climbing is useful for strengthening the joints, muscles and bones of the lower area of the body. It might seem difficult climbing stairs, but once you are used to the exercise, it becomes less strenuous on the body.

The chief reason that many find it difficult to climb stairs is simply because the body's strength is weak due to lack of exercise.

Be sure to stretch the body each time you begin to exercise, and after you exercise the body. Stretching provides flexibility and releases the muscles so they work at their best. In conclusion, swimming is a great source of exercise that helps support the joints. Swimming allows us to use the entire body, working it to a great fit. When we use the entire body, we are providing our body the strength it needs to reduce pain. If you cannot swim, you might want to invest in swimming gear that can enables you to flop hands and feet around in the water. This is a form of exercise and it does help. Again, stretches should be done before and after each exercise, and especially swimming since you wants to avoid cramping.

Various types of exercises can benefit the body in many ways. If you cannot afford the gym exercises can be done in the comfort of your home. With your music, playing you could do a few stretch exercises, by reaching up over your head with arms, stretch up left and stretch up right. Side stretches are simply and will help you earn fitness at the stomach area and the side areas. The stretches detail keeping the arms straight, while holding a cloth to help you protect the lower back. Stretch up right, front, left, and stretch up in reverse.

Now that you've done a few stretches do a few arm swings by swinging your arms behind your back while bending down toward the floor, bending down left, stretch up with arms extended over the head, and swing back the arms down toward the right again.

Now let's do a few elbow lifts by putting the elbows over the head and folding the arms so that both hands touch the elbows, stretching up, down, right, and to the side. Repeat until you feel the little aches that come along with exercising.

Next, we can do a few head rolls, knee lifts, elbow touches, forward bob, and elbow touch on the forward bob. Starting with the head roll, roll the head down to the front, to the right side, back, left side, and to the front again. Knee lifts; require lifting one leg up and touching the knee with the opposite elbow and repeating on the opposite side. Forward bob is similar to knee lifts, except you will follow the knee lift procedure, bob forward reaching half way to the floor, up again repeating the knee lift and back down in a forward bob.

Dance aerobics is one of the most valuable exercises to date. At one time dance seem to appeal only to those interested, but today everyone is learning to dance, since it was discovered that dancing is the ultimate exercise that works the entire body, and helps to control weight. To get started at home, you can start with the side steps. With your music playing, toss that left hip out to the side, twisting your body slightly in the direction the hip goes. Step front, step to the side, and step to the back, while you listen to the Boot Scooting' Boogie.

After finishing, do a few toe touches, rocks, shake it, jumping knee slaps, flick-kicks, and hip twists to work off those pounds. Be sure to finish with a few stretches and cool-down routines. Working out will not only builds those joints, it will protect your muscles and joints.

Strength Building and Body Movement - Grouping Muscles

Strength building is the practice that includes body movement at a steady pace to preserve a height of fitness and health. Numerous people combine exercise and diet together, however many fail to combine the proper diets and exercises that their body requires. A few people presume they need to isolate muscles to build strength. The truth is at what time the muscles become isolated the movements of the body do not work correctly. The body despite notions slammed around, work preeminently at what time its perfunctory portions are powering the vigor in motion.

Consequentially, this entails the large muscles to be in constant motion, which forces the smaller muscles in concluding a convoluted movement. Muscles work in groups, or pairs. For example, if the biceps are moving in one direction the triceps will move in the reverse direction.

At what time the biceps are in moving, the triceps are in a relaxed phrase. The progression is known as the opposed and/or antagonistic act of the muscle. Additionally, few people presume that sticking to a precise diet can build strength of the muscles, while keeping the body fit and trim. For instance, scores of people nowadays adheres to a carbohydrate diet, believing that this will help them to lose weight while preserving health. Contrary to their beliefs, the diet will not strengthen muscles, nor will it benefit them over the long run. In fact, new studies have shown that carbohydrate dieting alone will only cause harm to the body as the person grows.

To build and strengthen the muscles you must learn how the muscles work to goal toward precise training. The muscles not only work in groups, or pairs, rather the muscles also work slowly or rapidly in succession, moving in reverse building block procedure while utilizing power, and burst or boost the endurance of the muscles.

The climbing goals are the overall goal of obtaining achievement in fitness and exercise. The goal factors on movement and chemicals of the body. The large muscle groups assist the small groups of muscle despite the actions you do, yet at what time the muscles work in groups, the strength building course of action flows more effortlessly.

Swift moving exercises over short timeframes, thus the fast twitching of the muscles is not utilizing oxygen, rather the muscles are utilizing glycogen. When the muscles utilize glycogen, during workout thus, you are increasing speed, endurance and strength.

When the muscles slowly move, it is utilizing oxygen as the vigor, which the most frequent muscles utilized that powers oxygen is the legs, back, thighs, and hips. At what time you utilize the muscles ATP breaks down, thus manufacturing vigor. The disadvantage here, is that ATP breaks down more so in movements of the muscles at a slow pace, rather than swift movements of the muscles. Thus, the ATP in strength building must produce swiftly since it shapes a chemical response. To produce strength and power at a higher level, the pace enzyme arrangement must be active. Thus, combining or cross training is idea since you can use routines of aerobics that enforce oxygen, increase in enzymes and supplying sugars for fueling the body.

If your body is lacking fitness, it may take some time to generate the effect you want to obtain. Your body needs to adapt to the novel speed increase, fitness idea and so on. Most times, you will notice results in the first week that is if you continue the routine. You may lose a pound, but hey that is a pound you probably didn't need. Few types of cross training exercises work better than others training program. The overall idea however is to restore health while keeping fit and increasing the heart rate. If you are around forty years of age the idea, heart rate is around 155 according to few experts. Younger persons can get away with a heart rate of 140 while persons older than forty should work up to a rate of 130. Don't quote me on this, since this is merely coming from expert advices that were recorded in the early eighties.

Flex Exercise

Flex exercises are extremely significant to all of us, since flexibility assist the body, by responding to the way a person moves. Temperate workouts that embrace stretching exercises for increasing measurement lengthways of the muscles and motion of the joints, is a supportive source for gaining flexibility, and keeping the body's mobility unswerving...Stretching is not only exceptionally imperative preceding starting exercises, it is also central at what time a person sits or sleeps to long. For example, stretches are important when you get out of bed; stand from a chair, or after taking an extended ride in a motor vehicle. At what time a person stretches it aligns the body, stretching the muscles to eradicate soreness. Stretch exercises can consist of explicit particulars, such as upper thigh stretches, backstretches, leg stretches, and arm stretches and so on. Dance, yoga, and aerobics generally adhere to stretching, cool-downs, warm-ups, and so on before starting a routine. The main idea is to stretch the muscles to length, connecting the tissues that surround the fiber muscles. The action makes the body parts flexible.

After completing stretches, while participating in moderate aerobic classes, the trainee moves to flex motions, which comprise an addition few moments of stretching. Flex exercises brings benefits to trainees in a number of ways. For example, flex exercises will preserve the body's actions, while liberating motion. Flexibility also upkeeps the back and posture. Persons with history's or injuries that include back injuries should participate regularly in flex exercises.

Flex exercises also minimizing the odds of encountering injury, yet it is a great source for relieving pain from prior injuries. It is important to speak with your physician if you have injuries and/or prone to injuries before starting any exercises.

Exercise as a whole is excellent for relieving stress by relaxing the body. Exercises if done correctly will tone the body while building muscle structure. Flex and other types of exercises will help you control the weight, lose weight, and so on, yet exercise alone is never enough? Flexing aerobics or exercises are essential to enforce relaxation of the body, as well as assisting in mind power and physical relief.

Calf stretches can help you find a sense of relief. To stretch the calves you will need to place self in a standing position that feels comfortable to you. Put the hands on the hip area, before starting the stretching procedure. You can also place your hands on a wall to support self with the shoulders' apart at breadth. One in place, step to the front with the right foot about half the shoulder's breadth.

Bend the knees with both feet firmly gripping the floor. Shift the body with the foot extending outward, or to the front. Subsequent to finishing, lower the hips leisurely, until the body reveals mild stretch sensations in the calf area, or at the Achilles tendon area, which is the rear-left-leg. Continue the process on each leg up to fifteen or thirty seconds, per leg.

The stretches should be done first in my opinion. Trainers have their own idea as to what is correct, however the shoulders stretched before the calf stretching process starts can help you relax further. Standing with the feet flat to the floor in a comfortable position and with the fingers behind the back, palms facing the spine, and thumbs directing downward, hold you position.

Once in place, link the hands directing them toward the ceiling slowly, at the same time, keep the back and neck in an unperturbed site. The chest area should feel a sensation of stretching. The exercise should continue by holding in position up to fifteen to thirty seconds.

Personally, stretches done in the morning after getting out of bed, should be done lying down. Before getting out of bed stretch, the arms upward over the head and the legs stretched out at length. Stretch up with the arms and down with the legs as far as you legs and arm will allow. Repeat the procedures until you feel a relaxing feeling over your body. This in my experience has tremendously helped the lower part of my back, legs, and arms.

Chapter 8- The Benefits of Being Fit

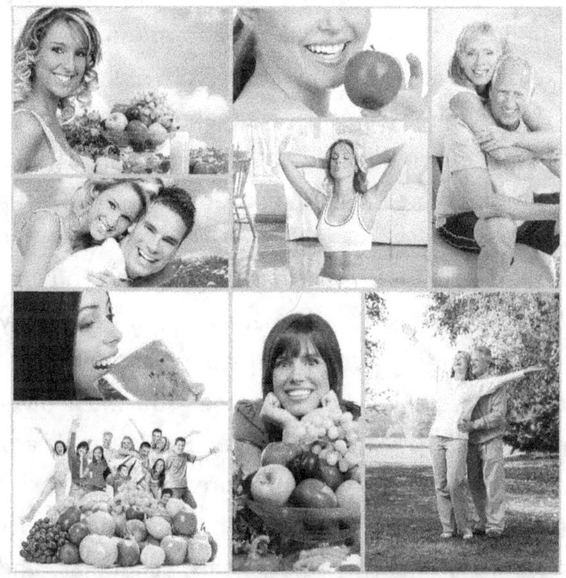

Did you know that you could live longer, stay healthy, and feel younger if you exercise and eat right? If you are eating healthy foods in moderation, and exercising every day you can feel good, stay young, and healthy while living a longer, more productive life. It doesn't matter how old you are, it is important to exercise regularly and eat healthy foods.

The Human Growth Hormones (HGH) is the source that controls the body's purpose. The HGH gives us the youthful look, strength, firmness of skin, high libido, and so on. The older we grow; the Human Growth Hormones ceases production. In order to maintain Human Growth Hormone levels, you would need amino acids, which "stimulate the pituitary gland in our brain." "The pituitary gland" enforces growth, "metabolism, and maturation in humans." This is only a part of where a healthy diet comes into play. Many factors decrease our health status and growth.

Our body requires a certain amount of Carbohydrates, Cholesterol, fat, calories, amino acids, and other nutrients to survive and keep us healthy. Yet diet alone is not enough to keep us healthy, make us live, longer, or keep us feeling younger. The body is a complex subject to understand. When we sit, lie around the house, or do minimal exercise, we are hurting our body, which increases our chance of feeling old. Lack of exercise and healthy foods is one of the leading sources why people suffer from heart attacks, strokes, diabetes, high-blood pressure, and other well-known diseases.

Diabetes is the MOTHER of all diseases and when you get diabetes; your health is at complete risk. It is important to avoid such complications by finding out which plan is right for you. There are three elements to staying healthy. One: You must divert a plan, adhere to a goal, and stick with the two. Setting goals are not hard for those that are used to the procedures, but for those of us that are spontaneous, setting goals can be a nuisance. The key to success is setting standards, rules, goals, schedules, and working toward making them come alive. If you have a spontaneous nature, then starting a planning schedule is easier if you write the plans down, and then put them in an area where you can see them each day. (Refrigerator, dresser, et cetera)

The key then to a healthier life is to plan a diet that is low in protein, cholesterol, low in fats, sugars, and high in fiber and starches. Your body will need enough minerals and vitamins to maintain a quality state of health. Some of the basic principles for starting a healthy diet plan are:

Starting with the body type and what your doctor recommends, try to include fruits, vegetables, small amount of meats and bread into your diet plan. Be sure to add bread to your diet. Eating two kinds of whole grain products per day can increase your health, and maintain your weight. Grains such as oats, barley, wheat, brown rice and so on are great for starting a healthy diet. Be sure to include raw vegetables, such as vegetable salads, cooked greens, and yellow vegetables. Potatoes include carbohydrates, so use this type of food in moderation, and avoid putting butter or sour cream on the potato. Fruit is another source of healthy foods. Citrus fruits should be consumed at least three times per day if possible. The expense of fruit nowadays if outrageous, so try to find produces that are inexpensive, and healthy: Fruit drinks are not considered a part of the diet. In fact, the USDA advises us not to drink a lot fruity drinks. Peas and beans are a great source of protein.

Protein should be used only in moderation. If you prefer meats, be sure the meats are lean and low in fat. "Low-fat, low-cholesterol animal protein" has Vitamin B12, and should be consumed and included in your diet at least once per week.

This is only a few details to help you get started on your journey to live longer and stay healthy while feeling younger, but it is important that you don't forget to include exercise into your plan.

Fitness and Exercise includes Nutrition

Fitness often leads to exercise and nutrition. In fact, you cannot keep fit if you do not exercise or abide by a nutritious diet plan. Fitness can take you too many places in life, but more specifically toward good health. At one time people walked to keep fit and called it there exercise for the day. Nowadays, millions of people are joining fitness and health programs where they participate in Yoga, weight lifting, aerobics, kick boxing, and other types of exercises.

Fitness is Sexy

Some of the most popular exercises today are aerobics and karate. Most health centers offer a variety of exercises to choose from, yet few health clubs ever talk about diet and nutrition. The larger exercising rooms offer loads of exercising equipment to the gym members; again, although the business is large they often fail to talk about diet and nutrition, which is a part of fitness and health.

Another part of fitness and exercise includes the face.

What does Facial Exercises Toning Include?

As we grow, wrinkles and crowfeet grow around the eye area, forehead, neck and so forth. Machines, creams, toners, and other natural care products can work to prevent wrinkles while decreasing facial fatty according to many.

Gels are sometimes the best solution for reducing wrinkles and restoring the face area to a youthful and healthy glow. However, the gels differ, therefore before deciding which gels is best for your skin, you will need to make sure the Gels purchased does not have chemicals that will harm your skin.

Pampering your face randomly, could lead to wrinkles, especially if you use products that harm the skin. Consistency is a great policy and procedure. Continuing to protect the skin will make room for healthy, fresh looking skin, while reducing wrinkles.

Masks

Masks employed tighten the skin about the face area, supposedly making the skin healthier while preventing wrinkles.

Facial masks and gels designed by Mary Kay are some of the better products. The products are not made from animal fatty as many other products are. There are no chemicals in the products that could hurt your skin.

Protective creams are sometimes good products, which help to keep your skin healthy and in tone while helping to reduce wrinkle. Some of the methods and products swarming the marketplace offer continuous resolution for wrinkle reduction, and according to many each of the products offer more than the other product does.

Facial Flex is different, since it provides tools, remedies, and solutions, which make the skin healthier, shinier, and helps to reduce wrinkling caused from aging.

Facial machines help to enhance skin and reduce wrinkles, preventing the wrinkles from developing. The facial machines have specially designed "pair of gloves." The machines include creams, which are employed to massage the face. The process helps to reduce wrinkles while enhancing the face and skin.

Facial toning exercises extend to pulling of the skin. Utilizing the mechanical gloves and applying the creams (lotions, gels, et cetera), will help eliminate wrinkling of the facial area.

Lines at the curves of the eyes are known as crowfeet. Crowfeet form around the eye area, accumulating from aging, narrowing the eyes, smoking, and excessive exposure of the sun. The apparent resolution is to avoid tanning beds, sun lamps, smoking and usual sun. Body weight can cause fat of the face, however if you continue to exercise daily you can avoid the unnecessary aging and deterioration of the skin.

Baby fat is widespread, thus using toners exercise equipment will help reduce the fat. Exercises include massaging the face area, wiggling the ears, moving the mouth in spherical motion, and so forth. Facial muscles lose tone when the area or muscles become too tight or too loose. Eating is one of the exercises for reductions, but eating unhealthy foods, such as fatties, saturated foods and are not, the better exercises to tone the face. Understanding all the details is the only solution available for toning and keeping the face healthy and youthful.

Ingredients for Poor Health Including Green Tea

If you suffer from infections or bacterial problems, (I would also bank on allergies after reading more into green tea history), then Green Tea can help prevent symptoms providing you are exercising and working toward fitness.

One advantage of including Green Tea into your diet and exercise scheme is that it can help prevent "Tooth Decay." Green Tea's "bacteria-destroying" capabilities reduce tooth decaying since it ministers to "the immune system with its anti-fungal properties by improving" the "digestive system."

Green Tea was originated "from the leaves of the Camellia Sinensis plant." Another advantage of including Green Tea in your diet is that the liquid drink helps prevent cavities. Imagine the money you could save by including Green Tea in your diet every day.

Green Tea ingredients combine EGCG with certain enzymes (DHFR-Dihydrofolate Reductase) to prevent cancer cells. Since Green Tea originated from leaves that are "steamed," this helps in the prevention of "EGCG compound from being oxidized." Oolong and black "tea leaves are not made from fermented leaves, which converts the EGCG into other compounds," that help fight cancel, infections, bacteria, arthritis, and other health issues.

So then, the Green Tea is the preferred choice to include in diets and exercise. Studies have shown that drinking at least 2 cups of Green Tea per day can help reduce health risks, as well as help with the process of weight loss.

Studies have also shown that combining caffeine with "green tea extract" helps burn calories, which enhances exercises that also burn calories. Researchers have found that drinking Green Tea offers an optimistic future for your health; however, you must not consider Green Tea as a source of the supernatural. Green Tea has been around for nearly five thousand years, and today its popularity is growing, estimating to be the second most favored beverage in households today.

Green Tea has three different flavors to offer, such as Oolong and Black Tea. The downside however is that Green Tea is fermented, while the other drinks are not. So therefore, if you are looking for health advantages, the Green Tea is in your best interest. Still, you must exercise and eat proper foods to stay healthy.

Carbohydrate Diet

Does the Carbohydrate diet plan work? To answer swiftly we can sum it up with a big fat no. The body requires a lot more than carbohydrates to work properly. The body requires exercise, protein, fats, sugars, grains, and other nutrient elements to make it work properly. These days' scores of people are going on Carbohydrate Diets believing that it is a fraction of the solution for upholding quality health, while staying fit. In fact, some people believe it is the only solution.

However, as the years' progress, losing or maintaining weight becomes difficult and health begins to show tale signs of negligence. During our growing years, the body alters along the way. Sometimes when a person grows, the body requires more than average, and will often crave different provisions. The body weakens during the aging process, and most times tires out sooner.

During the youthful days, it is essential to exercise and eat proper provisions to avert aging, and promote health while reducing the risk of illnesses. It is also important to avoid alcohol and drugs, or other harmful chemicals and substances that affect the body. Carbohydrate diets often lead to unhealthy living, since overtime the weight fluctuates and is harder to maintain.

While genetics play a role in health, including weight, it does not factor into what the body requires to stay healthy. In other words, if you are eating only carbohydrate provisions and not including other nutrients, the genetics will not make a difference in your health. Genetics is however a factor that determines the shape of the body, the weight, illnesses, and so on.

As we grow, the hormones affect the changes of the body radically. Carbohydrates are said by few experts to be one of the leading diet plans that promote health while losing weight. Yet, without exercise, any diet plan will not work to its fullest capacity. When a person adheres to carbohydrates without including exercise or other nutrients the body requires, as they grow they will experience headaches, dizziness, hunger and other symptoms.

Innovative researches conducted in the past few years' discovered that Carbohydrate diets can gradually make a person eat uncontrollably. Addicts of CARB diets are often perceptive according to few experts, since the rich provisions composing only CARB nutrients, lead to unhealthy living. Often the person endures unwarranted weight gain, which affects the body.

CARB comprise of sugar and starch. At the time it is digested, it goes to the intestines, which eventually lands in the insulin hormone and flows throughout the bloodstream.

Experts recently reported that the hormone insulin is one of the key elements that factor our weight loss or gain, and determines if disease are at high risk. The body must produce a steady level of insulin, before the body can work properly. As the body ages, insulin levels diminish the ability to produce other elements the body requires, such as chromium. Chromium is vital to insulin levels. Thus, confining self to CARB diets will only decrease the body's capabilities of controlling insulin, chromium, and other important nutrients the body requires to remain healthy.

The body demands movement to function properly. If the body is not in motion, it will gradually break. The muscles control the body's cells, tendons, nerves, bones, heart valve, and so on. If exercise is not part of the plan to stay fit, the muscles will gradually fail. The muscles control movement, heart valves, fingers, skeletal, legs, feet, and other parts of the body. If the muscles are weak, then the CARB diet is only diminishing your health.

As you can see, a diet should include protein, carbohydrates, fat, sugars, and other nutrients to remain healthy. Likewise, the body requires exercise ongoing to work toward reducing risks of illness, maintaining weight, and keeping fit without cease.

It is imperative to stick to a diet plan, but it is just as vital to work out. Before starting any diet plan or exercise make sure, you seek advice from your medical practitioner. Seeking his/her, advice will help you to avoid complications while starting exercises and diet plans. If your doctor tells you that CARB diets are idea, ask him/her about the nutrients the body requires, including fat, protein, and so on.

Cholesterol Fat

What does cholesterol and fat have to do with exercise and fitness? Many people assume that cholesterol is fat, nevertheless cholesterol is not a fat, and rather it is allied with fat. The body has both of these elements, and if there is, a deficiency or increase of one or the other, or even both it can affect exercise and fitness.

Cholesterol is varies of dense alcohol steroids, known as 'sterol.' Cholesterol is widely dispersed through plant lipids and animal meats. The substance is in wax form rather than in fat form. Cholesterol allies with fat, since cholesterol will not liquefy while touching blood plasmas or water. The body requires a level of cholesterol. The liver produces cholesterol in the larger quantity. The bile acids that help us to digest foods and liquids, and producing hormone steroids, including progesterone and GLUCOCORTICOID, require cholesterol production.

Thus, aerobics work with the cardiovascular muscles, which is important since increased levels or decreased levels of cholesterol can lead to problems, including ATHEROSCLEROSIS. The disease affects the heart, and is sometimes known as the Coronary Artery Disease. Thus, these arteries are the smallest cells in the blood, and they function to feed the heart's valve. Too much cholesterol then, will affect the heart, by hardening the arteries or narrowing the arties path line to the blood. Furthermore, excessive cholesterol will enlarge prostrates, since it converts to a form of crystal. Thus, cholesterol can cause artery disease if it reaches the heart and builds up excessively. The buildup of plaque reaching the bloodstream, affects the flow of blood, since it builds up forms of crystal while decreasing the flow of blood.

Excessive use of cholesterol narrows the arteries, and only trickles of blood flow through the veins and other areas of the body, which flows to the heart. This is why people have major heart attacks in some instances. This is also, why it is vital that aerobic exercises are entered into your life plans, coupled with adequate diet plans.

Collagen, cholesterol and fat make up the plague in the arteries. At what time the buildup occurs, the vessels are closed or isolated, and the tissues become reliant on blood flow, which leads to death of the arteries. Thus, higher levels of cholesterol starve the mind and body, and merely lead to strokes since the brain starves for oxygen, which is obsolete to a large degree and can lead to myocardial infarction. To determine you level of cholesterol add one hundred to your current age. Your doctor can also tell you the level of your cholesterol.

Lipoproteins are a substance in the body that carries cholesterol. If the lips are affected, cardiovascular problems arise, including disease. Pockets of fat are formed when VLDL or "very low density Lipoproteins" transfer from the liver a substance known as TRIGLYCERIDES. Generally, when a person eats too many sweets, fatty foods, or consumes too much alcohol the Lipoproteins are affected negatively. Thus, lips must meet a required level to maintain good health. HDL levels of Lipoprotein is essential for maintaining health, since the high dense lips level will clear superfluous residues of cholesterol, clearing it from the tissues, and sending the remains back to the liver where it is then secreted.

Now if you are still wondering what cholesterol and fat has to do with exercise and fitness, consider the body's requirements is a demand for staying fit and healthy.

Insulin also plays a part in fitness and exercise. When a person exercises and eats healthy foods, the body's level of insulin remains constant. If the body is lacking certain nutrients or has higher levels of particular nutrients, such as cholesterol and fat, thus the body's insulin is also affected. Therefore, learning what your body needs, what your body houses, and what exercises are best for your body is essential to reaching fitness and health.

The human body is never easy to understand. Yet, if we learn to understand our individual body, we have a chance to learn what is right for us, as well as learning how to stay healthy while exercising and eating right.

Maintained Fitness and Stayed Healthy

Anti-Aging, Weight Loss, Bones, Brain, and other issues that we face everyday... For example, your brain needs food too. If you are putting sugar and starches into your body, you are feeding your brain. Likewise, if you are putting any overuse of fats, calories, cholesterol, carbohydrates, or harmful substances, chemicals, foods, and so on into your body, your brain is affected... If your brain isn't working right, then your body likewise will fall short of your expectations.

If you are not exercising and eating healthy, then you can suffer bone deterioration, mental illnesses, chemical imbalances, aging, diabetes, and so many more health related issues that can gradually lead to death. Health and fitness is more serious than many realize. If you are not concerned about your health or fitness, then this is the wrong article for you to be reading; but I am not one of those people that take my health and fitness lightly. I don't go out and over exert myself, but I include some type of activity into my daily schedule. To help you see the importance of fitness and health, I am going to break down some medical issues so that you can see where negligence can lead.

Statistics has shown that one of the widespread causes of death is linked to "anorexia heart failure," and the widespread cause of death for "rupturing in the intestinal area as well as heat failure," is bulimia. I endured both of these eating disorders, and I am amazed that I don't suffer more problems that what I do now.

When we don't' eat right, including forcing anorexia and bulimia on our bodies, our internal and external body parts suffer. I can't stress enough how important it is for individuals to eat healthy. If you believe that not eating for days can help you lose weight then you are off balance. Sure, you might reduce your weight but you are killing your body and brain.

Most people are unaware that eating three meals per day in moderation can help them maintain weight, as well as lose weight. Eating right is part of your health and fitness plan, and if you don't know what you should do, the Internet, library, specialists, and other pieces of information are available to help you learn. Most of the information is free, so there is no excuses why you are not eating right, except that you are misinformed or simply don't care.

Fitness is Sexy

Bones are a part of our internal body that enables us to walk, run, sit, stand, and lift, and so on. When our bones are neglected because we are not exercising, then our bones are subject to deterioration, breaks, fractures, and so on. If on the other hand we are taking care of our body, then our bones will respond accordingly and walking, running, lifting, standing will not be a chore, but rather an enjoyable task.

Brain: Most people ask what the brain has to do with our body. Well the quick answer to that question is the brain is the core of our body. The brain has all our neuron, cells, and other components that make the bodywork. If your brain is not receiving proper nutrient, exercise, and so on, then your body will suffer. If you take a walk for example, your brain is recording this information. Similar to a computer, our brain takes in all data, activities, hardware, and so on and puts it in its proper perspective. If your brain is trained to a time where you are expected to walk as a part of your fitness and health, then your brain will trigger you when it is time for you to walk. On the other hand, if you are a couch potato, then your brain has no data to send, and therefore you will sit on a couch for hours, without activities, other than common worries and stress. That's right, if you are not exercising your chances of stress and worries are increased.

Therefore, put that body and mind to work and start your routine excise now to preserve your health.

Joint Exercise Preventing Arthritis

Arthritis is an 'inflammation of' the 'joints' and affects millions each year. The reason arthritis often affects the body is because it does not get the proper exercises needed to maintain a level of fitness. As we grow older, the chances of arthritis can increase, so exercise is essential for keeping our joints strong and healthy. Many exercises can benefit the joints, but for the most part, stretches are great for eliminating pain and strengthening joints.

Bicycling is a great exercise that can strengthen the joints. Walking, jogging, dance, and other 'weight-bearing' exercises generally strengthen the bones, but cycling is 'gentle on the joints' making it easy for all age groups to exercise with ease. Stretching is one of the better sources of exercises for 'strengthen' the 'joints.' Stretching exercises keep us flexible and reduces pain of the body. Stretch exercises provide us the best results when we stretch every day.

One example of a great stretch exercise is lying on your back in a comfortable area, with your legs extended at length and your arms above your head extended at length. Hold this position for a few minutes and relax. Repeat the exercise until you feel your body's pain decrease. Doing this type of exercise two or three, times per day can reduce body pain.

Static stretch exercises often focus to support the chest area of the body. The exercise procedure requires us to stand in a straight position with our 'feet slightly wider than shoulder-width apart.' The knees should be bent slightly, while our arms are stretched out 'to the side parallel and the palms of the hand facing forward."

Once in position stretch the arms as far back 'as possible.' To stretch your biceps stand in position with your 'feet slightly wider than shoulder-width apart." Keep your knees bent slightly, 'hold' the 'arms out to the side parallel' to the floor, and face the palms of your hands onward. Begin to "rotate the hands,' with the palms of your hands facing 'the rear,' stretching the 'arms back.' The upper backstretches require that you stand in position with your feet at a slight distance apart 'than shoulder-width, while the knees are bent slightly. Intertwine the fingers and then 'push your hands as far away from' the chest area 'as feasible. Allow the 'upper back' area to relax while in position. To stretch the shoulders stand in position with your 'feet slightly wider than shoulder-width apart.' With the knees bent slightly take our right arm and place it across your chest area, keeping your arm in a 'parallel position pointing toward the floor.

With your left arm extended up, use the 'left forearm to ease the right arm closer to' the chest area. Repeat the procedure on each arm. To stretch the shoulder area and biceps stand in position with the 'feet slightly wider than shoulder-width apart. Bend the knees slightly and situate 'both hands above' the 'head." Slide both the hands descending, reaching the middle of the spinal column area.

Repeat until you feel your body ease. Side bends are great for strengthening the bones. To begin stand in position with the 'feet slightly wider than shoulder-width apart," keeping the knees bent slightly while resting the hands on your hips; Slowly bend your body to one side, then upwards in position again, and proceed on the other side.

Be sure to keep the body from leaning forward or backwards for best results. To stretch the stomach and lower part of the back area, rest your body flat on the floor. Once in position, elevate the body from the floor, supporting the body with the toes and forearms only. Make sure your elbows are touching the floor and pointing 'directly below' the 'shoulders.' "Your forearms and hands should be resting on the' floor, 'pointing straight ahead.' Keep your 'toes and feet' at 'shoulder-width apart, while holding your "head in line with' the 'spine." After you have positioned yourself, 'contract' the butt muscles and hold the contract for about 'ten seconds.'

Next, you will 'lift' the 'right arm' from the floor, and 'straighten' the arm pointing it toward the ceiling over the head, and hold for '10 seconds." After you have returned to your position 'repeat' the procedure 'with the left arm' and then return to your position, lifting the 'right leg' from the floor while holding it for 10 seconds. It is important to keep the back in a straight position. Stretch exercises are said to be one of the great sources for strengthening joints.

CHAPTER 9- FITNESS: OVERALL WELL-BEING

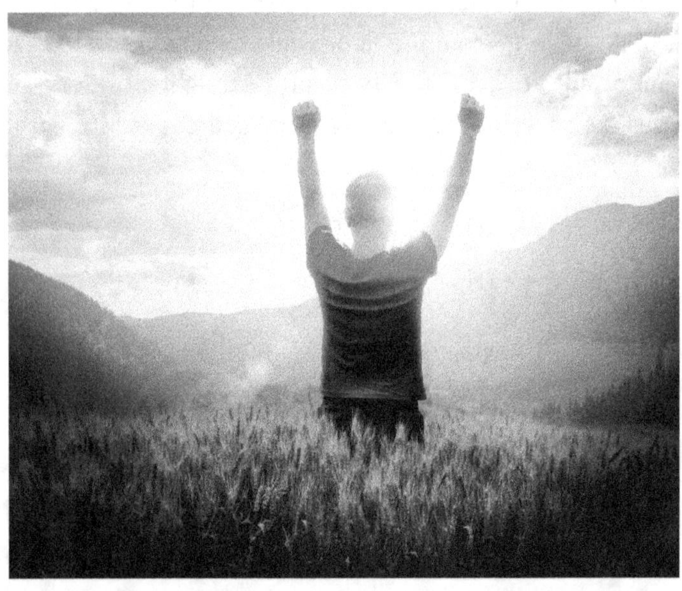

Some of the advertisement slicks claim that supplements can help build strong bones, while supporting health. The fact is, most supplements, recently was found to not have half the ingredients it claims to have. Thus, supplements are merely a pill with a price in most instances. The only way you are truly going to build strong bones and stay health is applying fitness and exercise to your life. The advertisements you often see are slicks that pull the wool over eyes, tricking you into believing that you do not need to do exercises or a adhere to a diet. If you have a diet system that works with your individual body, and an exercise scheme that builds bones, pills are unnecessary.

In order to feel decent and remain healthy the bones require motivation, support of the body, while working out daily. The body is a fundamental share we want to take care of to the highest aptitude.

The respiratory system and lungs supply the oxygen the body requires for breathing normally. Bones are indispensable, to endorse the lungs and respiratory arrangement. If exercising does not exist, the body will gradually deteriorate. Furthermore, if you are not exercising to strengthening the bones, then the oxygen intensity is pretentious. Consequently, aerobics is one of the better choices, since it influences and promotes oxygen. In fact, the expression aerobics derived from oxygen.

Many kinds of exercises boost the body's oxygen level and strengthening the bones, but the top respond is consider the body type to discover which exercise and diet plan is right for you. If you want to gain weight, the muscles and bones still require strengthen, so consequently put into practice exercises that work to develop muscle. The body comes in many shapes, sizes and forms, in spite of what shape, form and size you have, exercise is central to keep the bones robust and in good physical shape.

Exercise then promotes health and fitness. Now you ask how fitness bonds with the bones. Exercises are an indispensable, since it promotes health and strong bones.

Exercise makes the body feel good, while decreasing the aging progression. Exercise helps people to gain weight, lose weight, perk up health, trim down the risk of illness, while supporting the mind so it functions appropriately. Some people want to gain weight, still exercise is central. At what time the body is neglected, it has an effect on the cells, bones, tissues, mind, and muscles. It is vital then to plan exercise and diet plans that you can stick with.

To start exercises it is important to take it slow at first. Therefore, working the body up to 30 minutes of receptive exercise is a start. A number of the finest exercises that work to strengthen the bones are the 'weight-bearing' workouts. Weight bearing composes the right movements to burn fat, increase the bones and oxygen abilities, and so on. Some of the weight-bearing movements include, jogging, tennis, weight lifts, stair climb, walking, dance, hiking, and so on.

If you are heavy, then you may want to begin a workout routine starting with walking on a daily basis. You will commence to lose weight.

The concentrated workouts can advantage the body to a much deeper level. To build up the bones and muscles, working up to aerobics and weights is great. As you steadily expose the body to health, once you get into a practice, you want to boost the power of the workouts.

The bones are a critical part of the body. The bones help us to sit, stand, run, jump, and ride a bicycle and so on. If the bones are interrupted or weakened due to lack of exercise the bones can break, fracture, spring, become subject to disease and so. The diseases include heart failures, strokes, and so on.

With this in mind, if you are still asking why strengthen the bones you probably do not see a need for exercise which puts you at a high risk of disease and suffering. It is important to adhere to fitness and exercise to stay healthy.

Finding Weight

Losing Weight leads people to believe that going on a diet to lose weight is the ultimate choice; however many are unaware that exercise is needed to support their body's needs. If you diet to lose weight, you are not building muscle, burning fat, or enhancing your brain's functional capabilities. At what time you exercise you are feeding the brain, which in turns processes to the body. Doctor George Johnson at Washington University points out some confusion that is often made when people are attempting to lose weight, which I found interesting. The market is swarming with dieting tips, help, and plans to help people take off a few pounds. I often wondered about the plans, since each diet service has its own idea of what meals a person should eat to lose weight.

Thus, Doctor George Johnson says, "The fundamental fallacy of the Atkins diet, the Zone diet and indeed of all fad diets is the idea that somehow carbohydrate calories are different from fat and protein calories." The body's metabolism decreases when a person loses weight and increases when person gains weight. Therefore, the problem is Metabolism rather than calories and fats. When a person eats food that is geared to reduce calories and fat, it slows your metabolism, so therefore the person would also have to exercise to lose weight, build metabolism, burn calories and fat. When you include exercise in your diet plan, your body will need time to adjust. Therefore, when you are starting exercise it is important that you understand your body and its limits.

The best plan I found was to work out slowly at first. Be sure to do stretch exercises to adjust your muscles before you break out into a productive workout. Dieters should start out gradually and then build up to a productive full-body workout. Working out three times a week is the best possible solution for losing weight. Exercise should include aerobics (walking, jogging, et cetera).

Fitness is Sexy
Aerobic means "with oxygen," and the exercise works "the cardiovascular system," that "includes heart, lungs, and blood vessels."

Aerobics increases your oxygen level; at the same time, it involves the use of large muscles, which in turns "improves your level of fitness." After you get used to working out it becomes easier, and you feel better. You will discover your weight differences in a few weeks. Weight lifting on the other hand works to build muscle mass, while you lose fat.

Weights are great, but you should be aware that if you do not continuing working out with weights once you start, your body will flab and deteriorate, as you grow older. If you are only trying to lose weights, it is advisable to combine mild weight lifting with aerobics at least three times a week. When you first start out you should workout fifteen minutes per set, and gradually work up to a full-schedule workout, which usually lasts 30 minutes or longer, depends on you and your body. Now you can look into dieting. If you are doing aerobics and weight lifting, you should learn what nutritious meals could assist you in your weight loss program.

Green Tea is an excellent source for those of us that want to lose weight. Green Tea combined with caffeine is proven by medical experts to help reduce calories. Not only will it help you lose weight, it will also reduce your risks of cancer, arthritis, and other health related issues. One should also avoid consuming red meats, or eating too much meat. If you enjoy meats, then you should set a day aside that you will not eat meat.

In addition, you could add fish to your diet, as well as other healthy produces that will benefit you and help in your dieting plan. Hamburger is enjoyed by most people, but hamburger can cause weight gain. Avoiding meals that are cooked in grease then is another solution for losing weight. Cutting off the fat on meat, and broiling, boiling, or cooking them in water on top of the stove can reduce the calorie and fat intake. Dieters should be aware that breakfast is the most important meal of the day. Bagels, toast, or a light breakfast is always good, and will not affect your diet if you eat in moderation.

Reducing Stress

Reducing Stress with Fitness and exercise: Stress is linked to lack of Fitness and exercise activities. At what time a person avoids fitness and exercise the brain is affected, and stress is usually the result.

Laughter, Fitness, and Exercise: Did you know that statistics show that people who take care of themselves laugh more than those people that do not care for their health and body?

Avoid Meat as a Diet: Avoiding meat as part of your diet can help you reduce body fat, cholesterol, and so much more, according to few experts. However, the body requires cholesterol, carbohydrate, proteins, fat, and other elements to maintain good health. Before deciding on a diet make sure, you understand what your body requires before adhering to any diet.

Sleep, Health and Fitness: Statistics has shown that people who lose sleep will affect them, even if they are exercising, eating right, and taking vitamins. Thus, sleep is essential to reduce stress whether you are exercising and dieting or not. If the body does not receive the amount of sleep it requires then the body will show signs of suffering. New studies claim that the average person may require ten hours of sleep; however, throughout my years' I've learnt that the body is factored by the person. Your body will let you know what it needs, and your body knows more of what it needs than anyone other person in the world.

Weights as a source of Exercise Training: Many people are unaware that when they begin weight training, they must continue, otherwise the body is at risk. It is a fact that if the body starts a routine and stops or else stops and go changes of the body will occur. At what time you begin exercise the body requires a stable routine ongoing, otherwise, you may start gaining and reducing weight, or show other symptoms of negligence.

The fact is all of us need persistence to survive. If we as people do not have goals, plans, schedules and other necessities to keep us going, likely we will swerve along the path of life. The body functions the same as we do. In other words put your body on a schedule and stick with it otherwise don't blame your body when bad things befall you.

Diet Plans is essential to learn what plans work best for your body. Again, the body will let you know what it needs. You doctor may give you some advice but overall YOUR body is the one that will let you know exactly what it needs. Listen to your body talk so that you will know which direction to go.

If you are diabetes, or suffer, other medical conditions related you know that your body will lead you to problems if you digest loads of sweets.

Stress and stressors are a part of life. We all deal with stress and stressors; however, it is up to us to reduce the stressors, which lead to stress. The body and mind in fact provide you warning signs. If you fail to listen to those sounds, you will never know what your body and mind needs to feel fit.

The marketplace tells us about various types of exercises. WE have the Wall Slide, Dance Aerobics, Boogie Aerobics, Striptease Aerobics, and so on. We have weight training, martial arts and other types of exercise today. All exercises according to few will reduce stress, however the fact is if you are doing the wrong exercises you will add stress to your body. While all exercises offer something to all of us, not all exercises offer what we need individually. At what time you consider exercises make sure you listen to your body, since it will guide you to the path of understanding what is right for you and your body. If you are, starting exercises make sure you learn which diet is a better choice for your body. You will need to keep persistence in dieting and exercising once you start, otherwise the facts listed in this article will prove true in time.

No Substitutes

In recent days, an unusually large amount of advertisements slicks have promoted weight loss drugs on TV. They boast such things as, "lose weight while you sleep," or, "lose weight without exercise." As if there were some magic pill somewhere that could convert you into Vanna White or Charles Atlas while you sleep.

Not only is this notion ridiculous, but as any medical professional will tell you, any pill or drug you take will have some side effects that could be potentially hazardous. As usual, one should always consult their doctor before starting any new medication, or exercise routine. Nevertheless, there is no substitute for fitness and exercise.

Fitness starts with a good diet, which includes lots of fruit, vegetables and fiber in the form of whole-wheat or bran. I had always believed a good diet was important for many reasons, but like most people, I too, was unaware. That is until I saw a picture of a good friend that I did not recognize. As I knew him, he was a fit 155 pounds, full of energy and confidence. Little did I know he had a fat skeleton in his closet? He showed me a driver's license photo of himself taken just four years earlier weighing in at a whopping 260 pounds.

My friend began to tell me how he made his transformation. How he started watching his diet and doing exercises at home, bike riding, pull up's, sit up's and lifting weights. All this had him down to 190 pounds. Somehow, he couldn't drop his weight any lower. That is, until he read this article in a health magazine stating how the human body cannot break down sugar that has been bleached or flower. It seems that the body does not recognize the molecule after it has been bleached so it simply stores it as fat.

He began by cutting out all forms of white sugar. Of course, soda pop and suites of all kinds were kept to a minimum. He also began using whole-wheat pasta, bread and serial. He assured me, that it only took one month to lose 30 more pounds. I thought this was good information to have if you wanted to lose just a little weight.

Exercise also played a big role in his weight loss, of course. Many exercises can be done at home for the hard-core enthusiast. Nevertheless, if you're just an average Joe, like myself. You're looking for less strenuous ways to get in shape. Like long walks on the beach to flatten your stomach.

Alternatively, some yard work to strengthen the back and legs. In addition, for the cardiovascular workout, try some flag football with the kids. It's a blast. Volleyball is another good way of getting both the cardiovascular workout and working the abdominals. Any exercise in the sand will flatten your stomach. However, if you want to see results in a hurry, then I suggest you take up cross-country skiing. It combines the cardiovascular workout of jogging with the strength building of a stair climber. Watch out, it's tough but rewarding.

Some benefits that come with fitness and exercise are not obvious, but are still noteworthy. Benefits like, setting goals, and meeting them, building confidence in not only meeting your goals but also staying with your game plan. Set small goals at first. Such as, losing five pounds in the first month and as you meet the smaller goals, you can set your sights on bigger ones for the following months.

Either way you look at it, that person in the mirror, will only get better looking as you go. You'll find that the children don't wear you out quite as fast and that helping them with their Little League sports suddenly isn't such an inconvenience. Yes, the psychological benefits are there too, just waiting to be discovered. Besides, when it is all said and done, I'll bet that you will not want to trade your new body for old.

I have found that not everybody has to work out at Gold's GYM and looked like a Greek god. We simply should live healthy and be happy. In addition, it seems easier to be happy if you live healthy.

Overcoming Loss of Sleep

Did you know that many people are suffering from loss of sleep? Sleep is essential, not only for getting proper rest, but for functioning properly in our everyday life. We often overexert ourselves in daily schedules and work, which increases the stress level, making it difficult for us to sleep at night. When we are not sleeping well, it can lead, or even be a result of Chronic Sleep Disorders, Insomnia, or other medical related issue.

Some people find reading at night relaxing, while others claim that watching television in bed is a lead to falling asleep at night. Soothing music is also advised when a person has sleeping problems. The problem however is that your sleeping inconsistencies are not going away, since there is no resource for the body to function properly.

Lack of exercise and eating foods that are not healthy has been proven sources that causes sleep issues, including sleep disorders. Overworking is not a good idea. When you overwork yourself, you are only creating stress in your life. I realize life is hard at times, and sometimes we have to do more than we need to, but still we need a balance to function properly.

Few people believe that when they have a job that includes physical activities, that it is a source of exercise. The fact is, in most cases, it is not. Even if you have a job in the concrete or construction industry, it is hard work, but if you are not exercising and eating right, it could affect your sleeping habits, as well as your health.

Some of us require less sleep than, other individuals, but for the most part, we all require at least 7 or 8 hours of sleep to function properly. When we are not getting enough sleep, it affects us both mentally and physically. Lack of sleep affects our ability to stay alert, and process information. It also can cause us to have bouts of memory loss. In addition, it is not wise to work while you are tired.

If you lay concrete, or work with heavy equipment, you are putting yourself at risk and possibly putting others at risk. Depression can result from not getting proper rest. It can lead to violent behaviors, or other behaviors that not only affect you, but also affect others.

When you get enough sleep, you feel fresh, and motivated. If you have to consume caffeine to stay awake, you are only hurting your body further. Therefore, to get on the road to sleeping well, you need to divert a plan, set goals, and work hard to achieve them, by reducing your work hours, and increasing your exercise activities, and finding a diet that works for you and your body.

Caffeine (if consumed with consistency) is not a method for getting to sleep, and nor is it a method for taking care of your body. A well-planned diet consists of nutritional produces, liquids, and so on. It is important that you include fruits and vegetables in your diet, so that you are getting the proper vitamins your body requires. Once you have found a great diet that benefits you and your body, you will next need to plan a schedule where you can work out each day. Even if it is only for 10 minutes, at least it is a start. After about a week of dieting and exercising, you will start to notice results.

The results at first may be minor, but in the end, you will see the ultimate results and thank yourself for taking the advice to exercise and diet. It might be wise to include a Multi Vitamin regimen in your plan. In addition, if you consume alcohol you may want to cut back since it too can lead to sleep disorders.

Your REM sleeping stage is affected when you consume alcohol, and you do not get the proper rest you would, if you were not drinking. Alcohol also affects the liver, and the body. If you consume a lot of alcohol, it causes weight gain in some cases. While there are many reasons that sleep becomes an issue, most importantly when you are not taking care of yourself, you can't expect your body and mind to work properly.

Carbohydrates are one of the nutrients required in the diet, not to mention proteins and fat. Minimizing the nutrients is the key, simultaneously MAXING the plan you choose as your diet. The goal is to match the diet with your body.

Having too much of one nutrient in the body, obviously requires a decrease in the consumption of your plan chosen as your diet solution. Excessive CARB intakes in never healthy, and should be minimized for the better results. The disparity nevertheless, trainees attempting to mass-build require uptakes of calories to accomplish the goal desired. I'm not saying that eating more sweet is the answer; rather include in your diet added calories, more so than average. Sweets are ok now and again, however moderation is the ultimate option in anything we do in life to maintain, including maintaining fitness while living healthier.

Few drinks for health benefits can be added to your plan, since the body may shrink fastidious vitamins. It is important to stay away from harmful substances, including steroids. Steroids are extremely destructive, unless your physician prescribes the steroids as part of a solution for healing.

It is important that you visit your doctor before starting any diet solution, or exercise to make sure that you is on the right path to fitness. Medical practitioners often provided helpful tips, which could lead you toward fitness at a healthy pace, while building mass. Your general practitioner may advise you on which vitamins that your specific body lacks. Thus, including vitamins is essential when considering fitness.'

Supplements are disingenuous. Thus, banking on supplements to help you gain or lose weight, or else stay fit is only leading you nowhere, and it fact it could lead to harm since new evidence is claiming the supplements are detrimental. Keeping the body on top form requires training and dieting. Thus, take a look below to learn more about getting the start on healthier living.

About the Author

Sandra Hampton has been a certified fitness instructor for over ten years. She has worked with different types of people with different health problems, issues and insecurities. Sandra always put her mind and full support to her trainees to help them achieve their goal, which is to be fit and have a healthy lifestyle. Because of Sandra's experience and expertise, she is one of the most sought after fitness instructors in the West Coast.

Sandra and her family live in Sacramento.